the
REAL REASON CANNABIS HAS NOT BEEN RESCHEDULED

A CURE FOR CANCER DELAYED?

By Russell Redden

THE REAL REASON CANNABIS HAS NOT BEEN RESCHEDULED: A CURE FOR CANCER DELAYED?

ISBN-13:
978-1543166330

ISBN-10:
1543166334

This book was written in attempt to bring certain undeniable facts regarding the history of the Controlled Substance Act, and how this law has likely delayed the development of valuable chemotherapeutic agents—and epileptic and asthmatic drugs—from Cannabis.

This delay has possibly resulted in
hundreds of thousands of deaths
since Congress passed this law in 1970.

Sections

Introduction

A "Catch-22" series of regulations has been written into United States law, that has prevented a great discovery from being explored. Over 100 preclinical studies reveal that substances in marijuana can kill cancer cells, while leaving good cells intact. Despite these studies, the United States Government has failed to follow up on this evidence.

The scheduling system of the Controlled Substances Act is standing in the way of this research. Marijuana has been placed in a category that declares it has no medical value. The ability to move a substance from one "schedule" to another is next to impossible. The regulations of the Controlled Substance Act makes this change rare. This "red tape" has prevented research from taking place, that could possibly save *thousands of lives*.

Many people are alive today because they discovered these preclinical studies, and treated themselves with the concentrated oil of this plant, which has no psychoactive effects. These lab results reveal that both THC-*a* oil, and CBD (Cannabidiol) oil hold promise for the treatment, or cure, of various types of cancers. Yet, despite billions of dollars of tax money invested each year to find a cancer cure, our Government has not followed up this research with any *human studies*. For four decades, people have *suffered* and *died*, while a few researchers knew that a cure for cancer could exist in substances found in this plant. Men, women, and children, continue to suffer the ravages of radiation, and chemotherapy, while our government continues to invest in *other ways* to cure cancer—usually ending in *futility*.

If our government has been "sitting on" a cure for cancer for 40 years, it is a travesty, and an outrage. This book will present this evidence in a manner that draws no definite conclusions, only shines the light on the *irresponsibility* of the failure of our government to investigate. Furthermore, the *real reason* our politicians have not rescheduled Cannabis is not widely known. I hope this book educates everyone about this issue.

Change is difficult, but good people will rise to the occasion, once they understand.

Section #1
Cannabis as a treatment for various diseases, including Cancer

The placement of Cannabis in "Schedule I" of the Controlled Substances Act is a declaration by the United States Government that marijuana has no medicinal value. It also means researchers must jump through hoops of "red tape" to conduct human trials that would yield any *positive* results. Therefore, it is almost impossible to prove marijuana's medicinal value, because the Government has deemed it has no medicinal value, and stands in the way of any research that could prove otherwise. Usually, a researcher will be approved for a human, clinical trial only if he is trying to prove something *bad* about pot.

Many preclinical studies have demonstrated substances in marijuana kill cancer cells. Despite this evidence, the United States Government spends *billions* of dollars each year in cancer research into all *other* possible treatments, and cures. Cannabis *as a cure for cancer* has been virtually ignored by our Government for *four decades*, since the first lab results revealed this potential miracle.

The National Cancer Institute admits on their web site that substances in marijuana can kill cancer cells. We read:

'...groups of mice and rats were given various doses of THC by gavage. A dose-related decrease in the incidence of hepatic adenoma tumors and hepatocellular carcinoma (HCC) was observed in the mice. Decreased incidences of benign tumors (polyps and adenomas) in other organs (mammary gland, uterus, pituitary, testis, and pancreas) were also noted in the rats. In another study, delta-9-THC, delta-8-THC, and cannabinol were found to inhibit the growth of Lewis lung adenocarcinoma cells in vitro and in vivo ... In addition, other tumors have been shown to be sensitive to cannabinoid-induced growth inhibition. Cannabinoids may cause antitumor effects by various mechanisms, including induction of cell death, inhibition of cell growth, and inhibition of tumor angiogenesis invasion and metastasis.[1]"

THC, and it's non-psychoactive counterpart, THC-*a*, kills cancer cells in rats, and in test tubes. Yet, this is only one of many cannabinoids found in marijuana. The second most prevalent substance is CBD, or Cannabidiol. The National Cancer Institute also acknowledges that this substance kills cancer cells:

"An in vitro study of the effect of CBD on programmed cell death in breast cancer cell lines found that CBD induced programmed cell death, independent of the CB1, CB2, or vanilloid receptors."

The National Cancer Institute made these comments in reference to numerous studies that can be found on PubMed, the online database of the National Library of Medicine, of the National Institutes of Health. Both in vitro, and in vivo studies performed in many different countries reveal these facts. However, despite these studies, the National Cancer Institute also admits:

"**No clinical trials of Cannabis as a treatment for cancer in humans** were identified in a PubMed search; however, a single, small study of intratumoral injection of delta-9-THC in patients with recurrent glioblastoma multiforme reported potential antitumoral activity[2]."

Consider this statement. Their search of PubMed found *no* human trials, except for *one* small study. And, this study did *not* take place in the United States. This study was performed in the United Kingdom, and yielded promising results that THC might treat a rare form of brain cancer. Now, a company from the U.K. has applied to begin the *first* clinical trial of Cannabis as a treatment for cancer in the United States:

---

[1] https://www.cancer.gov/about-cancer/treatment/cam/hp/cannabis-pdq#link/_73_toc
[2] *ibid*

"GW Pharmaceuticals is already well on its way to winning the first-ever U.S. approval for a cannabis-derived therapy. But an early trial suggests that these treatments could also be an effective way to fight one of most devastating forms of brain cancers: glioblastoma multiforme. The U.K. based company unveiled preliminary data Tuesday from a mid-stage study on an experimental drug combining cannabidiol and THC, the "high" producing element of marijuana. Results so far show that the drug boosted brain cancer patients' median survival rates by about six months compared to a placebo. Typically, this type of cancer ravages the brain and (on average) leaves 70% of patients dead within two years of being diagnosed." (From: The Next Big Brain Cancer Drug Could Come from Marijuana. By Sy Mukherjee. Fortune Feb 07, 2017[3])

For many people who have Cancer, or who *had* Cancer, this news has come too late. The first study that revealed substances in marijuana could kill cancer cells was completed in 1974. From this study—partly funded by the National Institute of Drug Abuse, and performed at the University of Virginia)—we read:

"Lewis lung adenocarcinoma growth was retarded by the oral administration of delta9-tetrahydrocannabinol (delta9-THC), delta8-tetrahydrocannabinol (delta8-THC), and cannabinol (CBN), but not cannabidiol (CBD). Animals treated for 10 consecutive days with delta9-THC, beginning the day after tumor implantation, demonstrated a dose-dependent action of retarded tumor growth.[4]"

Two subsequent studies confirmed this in the late 1970's. They were published in literature released by the National Institute of Drug Abuse, in a report sent to Congress. Yet, our politicians did *nothing* about this news. It was buried in the static of the "news of the day"— while billions of dollars were invested in *other ways* to treat this deadly disease.

As stated, over 100 preclinical studies confirm that substances in Cannabis kills cancer cells, while leaving healthy cells alone. The appendix of this book lists these studies, with hyperlinks to PubMed, so that you can read them for yourself. It is amazing the various types of cancers that could be treated: pancreatic, lung, breast, melanoma, colon, brain, and leukemia to name a few.

[3] http://fortune.com/2017/02/07/gw-pharmaceuticals-marijuana-brain-cancer/

[4] Antineoplastic activity of cannabinoids. https://www.ncbi.nlm.nih.gov/pubmed/1159836

Yet, this possible cure for cancer has not been tested on *one* human being in the United States. Every year, dying patients who have no hope can try *other* experimental treatments, which in some cases, prove to be fatal. Cannabis has a safer protocol than many of these experimental drugs.

Despite lack of human studies in the U.S., these trials are beginning *in Israel*:

Preliminary Results From Israeli Study: Cannabis Delays Cancer Development
April 11, 2015
"Meiri and his colleagues have succeeded in causing brain cancer cells to "commit suicide," or apoptosis, a form of "programmed cell death." This is something a group of Spanish researchers has seen in the past, and Meiri has been able to reproduce it. One of the characteristics of cancer cells is their ability to evade the cell's mechanisms of death, and it seems cannabis somehow succeeds in putting this mechanism back into operation, even if the researchers still do not understand how, says Meiri. They have succeeded in producing similar results in breast cancer cells, and from there he wants to continue on to the other types of cancer[5]."

After four decades, other countries are beginning to investigate this treatment. If proven to be true, the obstructions placed in United States law regarding this issue will suddenly become macabre.

How many people have died in the last 40 years from cancer? How many men, women, and children have suffered? Eventually, if this proves to be a miracle treatment for cancer, the prohibition of the U.S. Government will suddenly become a bad taste in *everyone's* mouth. They will ask "why wasn't this investigated *years* ago?" and "why did the Government do *nothing* with this information, and let my mother, father, sister, brother, or child die in terrible agony?" These questions will be asked, and the United States will become maligned, unless it takes the lead on this issue.

Year after year, our Government has ignored this knowledge, while people *suffered* and *died*. The Controlled Substances Act has created this situation, by the placement of marijuana in Schedule I. Richard Nixon, and the 91st Congress created a law that takes the power away from the people, and places it in the hands of unelected bureaucrats—while it ties their hands to prevent any change.

---

[5] http://www.haaretz.com/israel-news/culture/health/.premium-1.651249

Medicinal Properties Admitted

The continued assertion by the United States Government that marijuana is devoid of medicinal properties is a farce. As early as 1977, the National Institute on Drug Abuse admitted to the medical properties of Cannabis. In their publication "Marihuana Research Findings: 1976," it is acknowledged that Cannabis can help with these conditions:

"Intraocular Pressure (IOP) Reduction

"Twelve open angle glaucoma patients were studied by the UCLA group (Hepler et al., 1976). In 10 of the 12, impressive reductions in ocular hypertension were achieved."

Bronchodilation

"Two lines of research, that of the Vachon group and the work of Tashkin and his collaborators, have clarified a number of questions about the effects of cannabis upon bronchial diameter. Vachon et al. (1973) observed the effects of a single administration of smoked marihuana on normal subjects and on asthmatic patients. They found that airway resistance decreased significantly in the normal group, permitting specific airway conductance and mean expiratory flow rates to increase. In the asthmatics bronchoconstriction was reversed for hours. From subsequent animal work, Vachon et al. (1976a) assume that the bronchodilation that follows -9-THC administration involves the adrenergic system. Recently, Vachon et al. (1976b, 1976c) used a microaerosolized -9-THC spray in 10 asthma This aerosol was found to decrease airway resistance by an average of 16 percent at 90 minutes and increase flow rates without any significant tachycardia or high."

Anticonvulsant
"Most of the work investigating the anticonvulsant properties of cannabis has been preclinical. The effects of cannabinoids on animal seizures induced by pentylentetrazol (Metrazol), audiogenic or electrical stimulation have been recently examined. Consroe and his associates (Consroe et al., 1973, 1975b; Consroe & Man, 1973) found that -8- and -9-THC blocked all three types of seizures in a dose-related manner."

Retardation of Tumor Growth
"Harris et al. (1976) have reported that mice innoculated with Lewis lung adenocarcinoma showed tumor size reductions ranging from 25-82 percent depending on the dose and duration of treatment with oral - 8-THC, -9-THC and cannabinol."

Antibacterial Activity
"In an effort to replicate the work of Kabelik (1957) and Krejci (1958) mentioned earlier, van Klingeren and ten Ham (1976) tested the antibacterial activity of -9-THC and cannabidiol. Broth cultures of staphylococci and streptococci were innoculated with varying concentrations of -9-THC and cannabidiol. They found that both substances were bacteriostatic and bactericidal, but were ineffective against gram negative bacilli."

Sedative-Hypnotic Action
"Sofia and Knobloch (1973) demonstrated that pretreatment of laboratory animals with -9-THC reduces the dose of barbiturates needed for hypnosis and increases total sleep time. Freemon (1974) confirmed the observation of other investigators that -9-THC, like most hypnosedatives, reduces REM time. However, in contrast to other hypnotics, the abrupt withdrawal of -9-THC after six consecutive nights of usage failed to produce a REM rebound, although mild insomnia was observed."

Analgesia
"Cancer patients in pain were studied by Noyes et al. (1975).

Patients were given either -9-THC in 5, 10, 15 or 20 mg doses or a placebo. Pain reduction was greater at all -9-THC levels than in the placebo condition. Significant pain reduction was noted at the 15 and 20 mg THC levels."

Pre-Anesthetic
"A number of studies have examined the role that -9-THC can play as a pre-anesthetic agent, with mixed results. When it was given prior to inhalation anesthesia, the requirement for cyclopropane and halothane was decreased (Paton & Temple, 1973; Stoelting et al., 1973). Smith (1976) found that normal volunteers given 200 mcg/kg THC intravenously experienced marked sedation with minimal respiratory depression."

Antidepressant
"A group at the Medical College of Virginia (Regelson et al., 1976) performed a double blind study with cancer patients receiving chemotherapy. An initial starting dose of 0.1 mg/kg t.i.d. was used. The dosage was raised only if previous doses were welltolerated. On a battery of personality tests and mood scales, the -9-THC acted as a mood elevator and tranquilizer producing significant improvement on two of three Zung depression scales. Cognitive functioning was unimpaired and appetite enhancement and retardation of weight loss were noted from clinical records. The need for narcotics was decreased, and patients had the impression that some pain relief resulted."

Antinauseant, Antiemetic and Appetite Enhancer
"The double blind Regelson study at the Medical College of Virginia is mentioned above in the section on antidepressant effects, but the researchers believed that the principal benefits seen in their cancer chemotherapy patients were the improvement of appetite and lack of the expected weight loss. Increased sociability and tranquilization were achieved by many patients according to the check lists used. Sedation, which could be desirable in this group of patients, was a frequent side effect. Nausea and vomiting were brought under control significantly more often by -9-THC than with the placebo."

Treatment of Alcohol and Drug Dependence
"Alcoholics became more angry and depressed after alcohol ingestion as measured by mood scales. Marihuana produced a

more positive mood state and did not interfere with the arousal reaction, although it greatly increased heart rate and produced an acute paranoid or confusional state in 3 of the 27 subjects. This investigator also found that disulfiram (Antabuse) and marihuana could be given safely together in the treatment of alcoholism. The study is continuing, but the early findings indicate that marihuana may be a suitable therapeutic adjunct for some alcoholics as a reward to encourage them to take disulfiram. Hine and colleagues (1975a) implanted morphine pellets in rats. -9-THC in 1, 2, 5 and 10 mg/kg doses were injected intraperitoneally 71 hours later. An hour afterwards, 4 mg/kg of naloxone (Narcan) was delivered into the same site. Attenuation of abstinence was achieved with a dose of 2 mg/kg and higher. Cannabidiol significantly potentiated the -9-THC effect on diarrhea and wet shakes. In a letter, Carder (1975) criticized the paper by Hine on suppression of naloxone-precipitated morphine abstinence. He pointed out that only two of nine symptoms were reduced (wet shakes and defecations). It was suggested that this could simply be a non-specific depressant effect . In reply, Hine et al. (1975b) stated that the decrease in wet shakes, diarrhea and bolus counts was dose related. The relative importance of one abstinence symptom over another is difficult to evaluate. Hine et al. retain the belief that a clinical trial of -9-THC in opiate detoxification is justified."

Consider how many people have suffered from these various ailments since this report was released 40 years ago. Since that time, many drugs could have been derived from this plant—safer than many prescription drugs, which kill *thousands* each year[6].

Since this report was issued in 1977, how many people have died from seizures? Asthma attacks? or by opiate overdose, attempting to treat chronic pain? Failure of our government to *follow up* on these discoveries—reported 40 years ago to the President and Congress—makes them partially complicit in these deaths. And, not only has our government *ignored this information*, but continue to make it a crime to possess this plant.

NIDA's report also reveals the anti-cancer, and anti-tumor effects of THC. We read:

---

[6] http://health.usnews.com/health-news/patient-advice/articles/2016-09-27/the-danger-in-taking-prescribed-medications

"...mice innoculated with Lewis lung adenocarcinoma showed tumor size reductions ranging from 25-82 percent depending on the dose and duration of treatment with oral -8-THC, -9-THC and cannabinol."

Lung cancer is a terrible disease. A possible cure was acknowledged in this 1977 report, and our Government did *nothing* about it. Consider how many people have suffered, and died of lung cancer since that time. How many people suffered the ravages of Chemotherapy, without any results? Sometimes chemotherapy works, but many times it only makes the suffering of these people worse, without extending the life of the patient. How can the government pretend to care about the well being of its citizens, and not explore a less toxic option? This is either evidence of incompetence, or a disregard for human life.

After this study was released in 1977, marijuana should have been *immediately* rescheduled. Why has this plant not been re-categorized? Various think-tanks, and medical institutions have stated that the placement of marijuana in this category hinders research. The National Academy of Sciences reports:

"Current challenges include the existence of certain regulations and policies that restrict access to cannabis products suited for research purposes (e.g., Schedule 1 status; regulatory approvals), the limited availability of funding for comprehensive cannabis research, and cross-cutting methodological challenges. Additionally, researchers are often unable to obtain the necessary quantity, quality, or type of cannabis product to address cutting-edge public health research questions." (The National Achedemy of Sciences. The National Achedemy Press. The Health Effects of Cannabis and Cannabinoids.[7])

The Schedule 1 status of marijuana creates many regulatory barriers, and has impeded research. These barriers were almost certainly *planned* by Richard Nixon, and lawyers in the 91st Congress who wrote the Controlled Substances Act. A regulatory nightmare was created, and this "red tape" has hindered science.

At the time this act was written, several warned that this law would hinder research, including Dr. Jonathan Cole, superintendent of Boston State Hospital :

[7] http://www.nap.edu/24625

"There is no reason to enact a bill like HR 17463. The bill would probably have no impact on illicit drug abuse... the bill puts all authority for drug control in the hands of the Attorney General and creates an inaccurate classification system. "High potential for abuse," the criterion for Schedule I, the most dangerous drugs, could be applied to food, alcohol, marijuana, cigarettes, cocaine, aspirin and amphetamines as well as heroin. "What really matters is not the potential for abuse but the seriousness of the consequence of abuse." Scientists investigating drugs would not have clear access to standard research drugs under HR 17463: "I see little reason to put special new controls on scientists or physicians just because drug abuse out on the streets is a big problem." (Dr. Jonathan O. Cole, superintendent, Boston State Hospital, testifying before Congress, representing the Committee for Effective Drug Abuse Legislation and the American College of Neuro-psychopharmacology)

This law does more than restrict the public from certain substances. This law places strict regulations on *scientists*, and *physicians*. Permission to perform studies on Cannabis have been limited for the past 40 years, as predicted by Dr. Cole. This "red tape" continues to this day, despite a *voluminous* number of studies that reveal Cannabis can kill cancer cells.

SECTION #3
The Controlled Substances Act

During the Nixon Administration, there was a great cultural divide in America. Many protested the Vietnam war, and many of these protestors had fallen prey to pseudo-Communist—or Communist—ideas. At the same time, drug usage was on the rise, and marijuana became the "symbol" of the hippy movement. In 1969, in a special message to Congress, President Nixon stated:

"To the Congress of the United States: Within the last decade, the abuse of drugs has grown from essentially a local police problem into a serious national threat to the personal health and safety of millions of Americans. A national awareness of the gravity of the situation is needed; a new urgency and concerted national policy are needed at the Federal level to begin to cope with this growing menace to the general welfare of the United States." (July 14, 1969, Public Papers of the Presidents)

Nixon continued:

"The Attorney General intends to begin a series of conferences with law enforcement executives from the various States and concerned Federal officials. The purposes of these conferences will be several: first, to obtain firsthand information, more accurate data, on the scope of the drug problem at that level; second, to discuss the specific areas where Federal assistance and aid can best be most useful; third, to exchange ideas and evaluate mutual policies. The end result we hope will be a more coordinated effort that will bring us visible progress for the first time in an alarming decade. These then are the first ten steps in the national effort against narcotic marihuana and other dangerous drug abuse. Many steps are already underway. Many will depend upon the support of the Congress. I am asking, with this message, that you act swiftly and favorably on the legislative proposals that will soon be forthcoming..."

Nixon called for a series of conferences, or commissions, to be conducted that would provide "more accurate data" on the "scope of the drug problem." However, Nixon placed emphasis on *one substance* in his speech:

"...These then are the first ten steps in the national effort against narcotic marihuana and other dangerous drug abuse..."

. There is an obvious reason Marijuana was singled out in Nixon's speech . Merely one month previously, the Supreme Court had just ruled in Leary v. United States. This ruling declared that the Marihuana Tax Act of 1937 was unconstitutional. Timothy Leary had successfully argued that the law violated the fifth amendment, which protects against self incrimination[8]. This supreme court ruling removed the prohibition of Cannabis on the federal level, and left its legal status up to each state. Without the Controlled Substances Act (or a similar law), individual States might have legalized Cannabis. This fact was likely in Nixon's mind, as he declared drug abuse as a "serious national threat."

Nixon introduced his bill, "Controlled Narcotic Drug Act of 1969" (f. HR 13743) in the House of Representatives, which proposed harsh penalties for marijuana, with mandatory minimum sentences of two to ten years. Many criticized this penalty structure, stating that the President's bill was a law enforcement measure, but drug abuse should be treated as a medical problem. After his bill

---

[8] https://supreme.justia.com/cases/federal/us/395/6/

was rejected, the House and Senate introduced their own bills, with input from the White House. The final version was the Controlled Substances Act, passed October 27, 1970.

The "Shafer Commission"

The Controlled Substances Act established a Commission to study the health effects of Marijuana. At the time it was established, many believed an "urban legend" that Marijuana caused violence. Since many Cannabis users were also protesting the Vietnam war, this appeared to be true—especially if there were clashes with the police. This misplaced fear of marijuana would be studied, as well as many other issues. Marijuana was to be *temporarily* placed on "Schedule I," until a final recommendation would be given to Congress a year later.

From the Controlled Substances Act, we read:

SEC. 601. (d)(1) The Commission shall conduct a study of marihuana including, but not limited to, the following areas:
(A) the extent of use of marihuana in the United States to include its various sources, the number of users, number of arrests, number of convictions, amount of marihuana seized, type of user, nature of use;
(B) an evaluation of the efficacy of existing marihuana laws;
(C) a study of the pharmacology of marihuana and its immediate and long-term effects, both physiological and psychological;
(D) the relationship of marihuana use to aggressive behavior and crime;
(E) the relationship between marihuana and the use of other drugs; and
(F) the international control of marihuana.
(2) Within one year after the date on which funds first become available to carry out this section, the Commission shall submit to the President and the Congress a comprehensive report on its study and investigation under this subsection which shall include its recommendations and such proposals for legislation and administrative action as may be necessary to carry out its recommendations.

While this commission was investigating these issues, the United Nations debated, and passed the Convention on Psycotropic Substances, February 21, 1971. The Controlled Substances Act was amended to be compliant with this treaty. The scheduling system of this treaty was similiar to the scheduling system of the United States.

At the same time, Richard Nixon—in several meetings recorded in the White House on what has been called the "Nixon tapes,"—attempted to influence the Shafer Comission, and prevent any recomendations that would include legalizing or decrimilizing Cannabis. From a transcript of the tapes, we read:

Richard Nixon: "When will the marijuana one come out?"

Shafer: "The marijuana will come out in March '72. In other words we are coming into the final phases of it now, we've had all of our public hearings. We have not, we have nine more informal hearings."

Richard Nixon: "It's now becoming a white problem."
"What you have here is a very interesting live situation, where there is a certain [unintelligible] through the country, that, heh, on the one hand want to make smoking illegal, cigarette smoking illegal and marijuana legal. Now, that's what I mean, that doesn't make any damned sense now. I mean, probably if we repeat what that didn't help its best aspects everything shouldn't do anything shouldn't need it, but uh, you know if they're going to [unintelligible]. On the marijuana thing, I have very strong feelings that that's, uh the, best final, uh, analysis, that once you start down that road, uh, the chances of going further down that road are greater. I'm aware some disagree with that, but uh, the uh, and also we have some people that are, frankly promoting it. They're not good people."

Richard Nixon in these tapes expressed a racist attitude concerning marijuana. He believed it was a problem among African Americans, and Hispanics, but was now becoming a "white problem." Regarding people who smoke Cannabis, Nixon commented, "they're not good people." This echoes the words of Jeff Sessions, who stated "good people do not smoke marijuana." This is a stereotypical view of the drug. Compared to how people act on alcohol, marijuana is benign. This was exactly the view of the Shafer Commission in their report, titled "Marijuana: A signal of Misunderstanding." It stated that marijuana does not cause violence, and should be decriminalized:

"The total prohibition scheme was rejected primarily because no sufficiently compelling social reason, predicated on existing knowledge, justifies intrusion by the criminal justice system into the private lives of individuals who use marihuana. The Commission is of the unanimous opinion that marihuana use is not such a grave problem that individuals who smoke marihuana, and possess it for that purpose, should be subject to criminal procedures. On the other hand, we have also rejected the regulatory or legalization scheme because it would institutionalize availability of a drug which has uncertain long-term effects and which may be of transient social interest.

Instead we recommend a partial prohibition scheme which we feel has the following benefits:

Symbolizing a continuing societal discouragement of use;

Facilitating the deemphasis of marihuana essential to answering dispassionately so many of the unanswered questions;

Permitting a simultaneous medical, educational, religious, and parental effort to concentrate on reducing irresponsible use and remedying its consequences;

Removing the criminal stigma and the threat of incarceration from a widespread behavior (possession for personal use) which does not warrant such treatment;

Relieving the law enforcement community of the responsibility for enforcing a law of questionable utility, and one which they cannot fully enforce, thereby allowing concentration on drug trafficking and crimes against persons and property;

Relieving the judicial calendar of a large volume of marihuana possession cases which delay the processing of more serious cases; and

Maximizing the flexibility of future public responses as new information comes to light.

No major change is required in existing law to achieve all of these benefits. In general, we recommend only a decriminalization of possession of marihuana for personal use on both the state and federal levels. The major features of the recommended scheme are that: production and distribution of the drug would remain criminal activities as would possession with intent to distribute commercially; marihuana would be contraband subject to confiscation in public places; and criminal sanctions would be withdrawn from private use and possession incident to such use, but, at the state level, fines would be imposed for use in public[9]."

Richard Nixon rejected these recommendations, which would have removed Marijuana from "Schedule 1." Instead, Cannabis remained in this Schedule, a declaration of no medicinal properties. It has been kept in this Schedule *year* after *year* by bureaucrats, who use red tape to deny a speedy hearing to the petitioners. Furthermore, a "Catch-22" provision in this law makes moving this drug to a different Schedule almost impossible.

The Attorney General Has the Power

During his confirmation hearing, Attorney General Jeff Sessions stated this about the laws regarding marijuana in the United States:

"One obvious concern is that Congress has made the possession of marijuana in every state an illegal act. If that is not desired any longer, Congress should pass a law to change it. It's not the attorney general's job to decide which laws to enforce. We should enforce the laws as effectively as we are able."

Senator Sessions obviously had not read the Controlled Substances Act. The responsibility to reschedule marijuana is given

---

[9] http://www.druglibrary.org/schaffer/library/studies/nc/ncrec1_11.htm

to the *Attorney General, not* Congress. From the Controlled Substances Act, we read:

> SEC. 201. [21 U.S.C. 811] (a) The Attorney General shall apply the provisions of this title to the controlled substances listed in the schedules established by section 202 of this title and to any other drug or other substance added to such schedules under this title. Except as provided in subsections (d) and (e), the Attorney General may by rule—(1) add to such a schedule or transfer between such schedules any drug or other substance if he—
> (A) finds that such drug or other substance has a potential for abuse, and
> (B) <u>makes with respect to such drug or other substance the findings prescribed by subsection (b) of section</u>
> <u>202 for the schedule in which such drug is to be placed</u>; or
> (2) <u>remove any drug or other substance from the schedules if he finds that the drug or other substance does not meet the requirements for inclusion in any schedule</u>. Rules of the Attorney General under this subsection shall be made on the record after opportunity for a hearing pursuant to the rulemaking procedures prescribed by subchapter II of chapter 5 of title 5 of the United States Code. <u>Proceedings for the issuance, amendment, or repeal of such rules may be initiated by the Attorney General (1) on his own motion, (2) at the request of the Secretary, or (3) on the petition of any interested party</u>.

The *Attorney General* has the power under this law to reschedule a substance. Proceedings to reschedule a drug can be initiated by the Attorney General, the Secretary of Health, Education and Welfare, or an "interested party." The term "interested party" appears to provide a voice to the average citizen, enabling them to petition their government to reschedule any substance. As we continue to read, we discover that the Secretary of Health, Education, and Welfare[10] can overrule the Attorney General, in his Scheduling decisions:

> The recommendations of the Secretary to the Attorney General shall be binding on the Attorney General as to such scientific and medical matters, and if the Secretary recommends that a

---

[10] Called the Secretary of Health and Human Services today

drug or other substance not be controlled, the Attorney General shall not control the drug or other substance. (SEC. 201. b)

It *appears* the Controlled Substances Act places science, and health, above Law enforcement. The Secretary of Health, Education, and Welfare has the power to overrule the Attorney General, if he recommends a drug "not be controlled." Yet this is a trick, and subterfuge. Many laws, or regulations in section 201 are rendered *meaningless*, by a "catch-22," or double-blind written into this law. I believe the lawyers of the 91st Congress— and Richard Nixon, who was also a lawyer—wrote these conflicting laws *on purpose*.

The words we have just read appear to answer the critics of Nixon's first bill, which was a law enforcement measure. In the Controlled Substances Act, the person in charge of *health* (the Secretary of Health, Education, and Welfare,) can override the person in charge of the law. And, these regulations allow a private citizen to petition their government. This *sounds* fair. However, it was meant to seem that way. As we continue to read, we discover:

"Sec 201 (d)(1) If control is required by United States obligations **under international treaties, conventions, or protocols** in effect on the effective date of this part, **the Attorney General shall issue an order controlling such drug under the schedule he deems most appropriate to carry out such obligations**, without regard to the findings required by subsection (a) of this section or section 202(b) and without regard to the procedures prescribed by subsections (a) and (b) of this section."

The Attorney General *must* keep the obligations of "international treaties" in his decision, **"without regard to the procedures prescribed by subsections (a) and (b) of this section."** The procedures prescribed by subsections (a) and (b) are those that give the Attorney General authority to reschedule a substance; those that give the Secretary of Health, Education, and Welfare the power to overrule the Attorney General's decision; and power to petition the government to any "interested party." All of these vital procedures, and laws are *annulled* by the words of section 201 (d). The Attorney General is constrained by the obligations of international treaties. These obligations are placed before or above the right of the people to petition their government; or any decision made by the Attorney General himself; or the Secretary of Health, Education, and Welfare.

As we continue to read, we discover that the power of the Attorney General to reschedule a drug is dependent on the decisions of the *Secretary General of the United Nations*, and the *World Health Organization*:

"Whenever the Secretary of State receives notification from the Secretary-General of the United Nations that information has been transmitted by or to the World Health Organization, pursuant to article 2 of the Convention on Psychotropic Substances, which may justify adding a drug or other substance to one of the schedules of the Convention, transferring a drug or substance from one schedule to another, or deleting it from the schedules, the Secretary of State shall immediately transmit the notice to the Secretary of Health, Education, and Welfare who shall publish it in the Federal Register and provide opportunity to interested persons to submit to him comments respecting the scientific and medical evaluations which he is to prepare respecting such drug or substance. The Secretary of Health, Education, and Welfare shall prepare for transmission through the Secretary of State to the World Health Organization such medical and scientific evaluations as may be appropriate regarding the possible action that could be proposed by the World Health Organization respecting the drug or substance with respect to which a notice was transmitted under this subparagraph. (B) Whenever the Secretary of State receives information that the Commission on Narcotic Drugs of the United Nations proposes to decide whether to add a drug or other substance to one of the schedules of the Convention, transfer a drug or substance from one schedule to another, or delete it from the schedules, the Secretary of State shall transmit timely notice to the Secretary of Health, Education, and Welfare of such information who shall publish a summary of such information in the Federal Register and provide opportunity to interested persons to submit to him comments respecting the recommendation which he is to furnish, pursuant to this subparagraph, respecting such proposal. The Secretary of Health, Education, and Welfare shall evaluate the proposal and furnish a recommendation to the Secretary of State which shall be binding on the representative of the United States in discussions and negotiations relating to the proposal. (3) 19 When the United States receives notification of a scheduling decision pursuant to article 2 of the Convention on Psychotropic Substances that a drug or other substance has been added or transferred to a schedule specified in the notification or receives notification (referred to in this subsection as a "schedule notice") that existing legal controls applicable under this title to a drug or substance and the controls required by the Federal Food, Drug, and Cosmetic Act do not meet the requirements of the schedule of the Convention in which such drug or substance has been placed, the Secretary of Health, Education, and Welfare, after consultation with the Attorney General, shall first determine whether existing legal controls under this title applicable to the drug or substance and the controls required by the Federal Food, Drug, and Cosmetic Act, meet the requirements of the schedule specified in the notification or schedule notice and shall take the following action: (A) If such requirements are met by such existing controls but the Secretary of Health, Education, and Welfare nonetheless believes that more stringent controls should be applied to the drug or substance, the Secretary shall recommend to the Attorney General that he initiate proceedings for scheduling the drug or substance, pursuant to subsections (a) and (b) of this section, to apply to such controls. (B) If such requirements are not met by such existing controls and the Secretary of Health, Education, and Welfare concurs in the scheduling decision or schedule notice transmitted by the notification, the Secretary shall recommend to the Attorney General that he initiate proceedings for scheduling the drug or substance under the appropriate schedule pursuant to subsections (a) and (b) of this section, to apply such additional controls; (ii) request the Secretary of State to transmit a notice of qualified acceptance, within the period specified in the Convention, pursuant to paragraph 7 of article 2 of the Convention, to the Secretary-General of the United Nations; (iii) request the Secretary of State to transmit a notice of qualified acceptance as prescribed in clause (ii) and request the Secretary of State to ask for a review by the Economic and Social Council of the United Nations, in accordance with paragraph 8 of article 2 of the Convention, of the scheduling decision; or (iv) in the case of a schedule notice, request the Secretary of State to take appropriate action under the Convention to initiate proceedings to remove the drug or substance from the schedules under the Convention or to transfer the drug or substance to a schedule under the Convention different from the one specified in the schedule notice. " (201, 2b, 3)

These paragraphs state that the decision to reschedule a drug depends on how that drug is scheduled in *the Convention on Psychotropic Substances*. When the Controlled Substances Act was passed in 1970, the international treaty the Attorney General had to honor was the United Nations Single Convention on Narcotic Drugs[11]. However, the Convention on Psychotropic Substances was passed one year later (which has a similar scheduling system as the United States.) The Controlled Substances Act was amended to comply with this treaty. In this treaty, there are procedures in place that puts the United Nations in charge of scheduling decisions, and international laws regarding the regulation of drugs, which all nations that signed this treaty must obey. The Controlled Substances Act was amended to follow the procedures of Paragraph 7, article 2, of the U.N. treaty:

7. Any decision of the Commission taken pursuant to this article shall be communicated by the Secretary-General to all States Members of the United Nations, to non-member States Parties to this Convention, to the World Health Organization and to the Board. Such decision shall become fully effective with respect to each Party 180 days after the date of such communication, except for any Party which, within that period, in respect of a decision adding a substance to a Schedule, has transmitted to the Secretary-General a written notice that, in view of exceptional circumstances, it is not in a position to give effect with respect to that substance to all of the provisions of the Convention applicable to substances in that Schedule. Such notice shall state the reasons for this exceptional action. (Article 2, paragraph 7, the United Nations Convention on Psycotropic Substances, 1971)

---

[11] Treaty passed, March 30, 1961

The removal of a drug from a schedule, or to a different schedule, begins with the communication from the Attorney General or the Secretary of Health, Education, and Welfare, through the Secretary of State to the Secretary General of the United Nations, who communicates with the World Health Organization. If an agreement is achieved, the decision is then transmitted to every individual nation state.

These are the procedures of "red tape" that has kept Cannabis illegal *worldwide*—and could be keeping a cure for cancer from being used by your doctor, or through self-administration.

If the Attorney General does not follow the scheduling system of the U.N., he breaks an international treaty, and therefore breaks the law according to the Controlled Substances Act. Seven years after the Convention on Psychotropic Substances treaty was signed, Jimmy Carter signed the *United States* Psychotropic Substances Act, which further stipulates that the United States *must honor international treaties* regarding drug laws. From the footnotes of this law, we read:

(1) The Congress has long recognized the danger involved in the manufacture, distribution, and use of certain psychotropic substances for nonscientific and nonmedical purposes, and has provided strong and effective legislation to control illicit trafficking and to regulate legitimate uses of psychotropic substances in this country. Abuse of psychotropic substances has become a phenomenon common to many countries, however, and is not confined to national borders. It is, therefore, essential that the United States cooperate with other nations in establishing effective controls over international traffic in such substances.

(2) The United States has joined with other countries in executing an international treaty, entitled the Convention on Psychotropic Substances and signed at Vienna, Austria, on February 21, 1971, which is designed to establish suitable controls over the manufacture, distribution, transfer, and use of certain psychotropic substances. The Convention is not self-executing, and the obligations of the United States thereunder may only be performed pursuant to appropriate legislation. It is the intent of the Congress that the amendments

made by this Act, together with existing law, will enable the United States to meet all of its obligations under the Convention and that no further legislation will be necessary for that purpose. (21 U.S.C. § 801a)

This law further ties the drug laws of the United States to the U.N. Convention on Psychotropic Substances. These laws that bind the actions of the United States to international drug treaties have prevented any reform of marijuana law. International agreements must be followed. This is the *real reason* marijuana has remained on Schedule 1.

Richard Nixon, and the 91st Congress created a "Catch-22" system of regulations in the Controlled Substances Act, which in the end binds the decisions of the Attorney General to the regulations of the United Nations. Only if the U.N. reschedules a drug, can the Attorney General reschedule a drug in the United States. The Secretary of State must go to the United Nations, and any rescheduling cleared through the World Health Organization— before the Attorney General *really* has the authority to reschedule a substance.

The Attorney General can schedule a drug *higher* than the Scheduling system of the U.N.

Although the Attorney General is bound to follow the Scheduling system of the United Nations if a drug or substance is removed from a Schedule—or rescheduled—he can Schedule that drug in a category *higher* than the Convention on Psycotropic Substances. From the Controlled Substances Act, we read:

(3) 19 When the United States receives notification of a scheduling decision pursuant to article 2 of the Convention on Psychotropic Substances that a drug or other substance has been added or transferred to a schedule specified in the notification or receives notification (referred to in this subsection as a "schedule notice") that existing legal controls applicable under this title to a drug or substance and the controls required by the Federal Food, Drug, and Cosmetic Act **do not meet the requirements of the schedule of the Convention in which such drug or substance has been placed**, the Secretary of Health, Education, and Welfare, after

consultation with the Attorney General, shall first determine whether existing legal controls under this title applicable to the drug or substance and the controls required by the Federal Food, Drug, and Cosmetic Act, meet the requirements of the schedule specified in the notification or schedule notice and shall take the following action: (A) If such requirements are met by such existing controls but the **Secretary of Health, Education, and Welfare nonetheless believes that more stringent controls should be applied to the drug or substance,** the Secretary shall recommend to the Attorney General that he initiate proceedings for scheduling the drug or substance, pursuant to subsections (a) and (b) of this section, to apply to such controls.

(B) If such requirements are not met by such existing controls and the Secretary of Health, Education, and Welfare concurs in the scheduling decision or schedule notice transmitted by the notification, the Secretary shall recommend to the Attorney General that he initiate proceedings for scheduling the drug or substance under the appropriate schedule pursuant to subsections (a) and (b) of this section.

(C) If such requirements are not met by such existing controls and the Secretary of Health, Education, and Welfare does not concur in the scheduling decision or schedule notice transmitted by the notification, the Secretary shall— (i) **if he deems that additional controls are necessary to protect the public health and safety**, recommend to the Attorney General that he initiate proceedings for scheduling the drug or substance pursuant to subsections (a) and (b) of this section, **to apply such additional controls**; (ii) request the Secretary of State to transmit a notice of qualified acceptance, within the period specified in the Convention, to the Secretary-General of the United Nations; (iii) request the Secretary of State to transmit a notice

of qualified acceptance as prescribed in clause (ii) and request the Secretary of State to ask for a review by the Economic and Social Council of the United Nations, in accordance with paragraph 8 of article 2 of the Convention, of the scheduling decision; or (iv) in the case of a schedule notice, request the Secretary of State to take appropriate action under the Convention to initiate proceedings to remove the drug or substance from the schedules under the

Convention or to transfer the drug or substance to a schedule under the Convention different from the one specified in the schedule notice."

If the United Nations transfers a drug to a different schedule in the Convention on Psycotropic Substances, but the Attorney General, or the Secretary of Health, Education, and Welfare believes additional controls are necessary, they can apply these controls under subsections (a) or (b). These were the subsections *made void* if "international treaties" must be followed. However, they become valid if United States officials *believe* additional controls are needed to "protect public safety."

These procedures allow the placement of a drug in a higher schedule, but also direct the Secretary of State to initiate proceedings in the U.N. to reschedule the drug, according to paragraph 8, article 2 of the Convention on Psycotropic Substances:

8. a) The decisions of the Commission taken under this article shall be subject to review by the Council upon the request of any Party filed within 180 days from receipt of notification of the decision. The request for review shall be sent to the Secretary-General together with all relevant information upon which the request for review is based.
b) The Secretary-General shall transmit copies of the request for review and the relevant information to the Commission, to the World Health Organization and to all the Parties, inviting them to submit comments within ninety days. All comments received shall be submitted to the Council for consideration.
c) The Council may confirm, alter or reverse the decision of the Commission. Notification of the Council's decision shall be transmitted to all States Members of the United Nations, to non-member States Parties to this Convention, to the Commission, to the World Health Organization and to the Board.
d) During pendency of the review, the original decision of the Commission shall, subject to paragraph 7, remain in effect.

All these laws describe a maze of both national, and international laws, designed to allow the politicians of America to derail the legalization of Cannabis. The Attorney General, or the Secretary of Health, Education, and Welfare, *must* keep international treaties, and schedules similar to the Convention on Psychotropic Substances—unless there is a fear of "public harm," then a substance can be placed in a *higher* schedule, without U.N. "approval."

Recent Warnings of the United Nations

The United Nations has warned the United States that the legalization of Cannabis in Colorado and Washington violate international agreements:

UN drugs body warns US states and Uruguay over cannabis legalisation
The Guardian, March 3, 2015
"The United Nations has renewed its warnings to Uruguay and the US states of Colorado and Washington that their cannabis legalisation policies fail to comply with international drug treaties.
The annual report from the UN's International Narcotics Control Board, which is responsible for policing the drug treaties, said it would send a high-level mission to Uruguay, which became the first country to legalise the production, distribution, sale and consumption of cannabis for recreational purposes.
The UN drug experts said they would also continue their dialogue with the US government over the commercial sale and distribution of cannabis in Colorado and Washington state.[12]"

One year later, the United Nations warned Canada about the legalization of marijuana:

---

[12] https://www.theguardian.com/society/2015/mar/03/un-drugs-body-warns-us-states-and-uruguay-over-cannabis-legalisation

Legalizing pot in Canada will run afoul of global treaties, Trudeau warned
Trudeau's plan to legalize, regulate and restrict access to marijuana complicated by treaty obligations
CBC News, Jan 5, 2016

"The Liberal government will have to do substantial work on the international stage before it can follow through on Prime Minister Justin Trudeau's promise to legalize marijuana, new documents suggest. That work will have to include figuring out how Canada would comply with three international treaties to which the country is a party, all of which criminalize the possession and production of marijuana.[13]"

The National Academy of Sciences has reported this fact about the Controlled Substances Act:

"Today, cannabis is regulated by local, state, federal, and international law. State laws often mirror federal law, enshrined in the Comprehensive Drug Abuse Prevention and Control Act of 1970, which includes the Controlled Substances Act (CSA). The CSA modernized and consolidated earlier federal drug laws, making them consistent with international drug control conventions, specifically the United Nations Single Convention on Narcotic Drugs of 1961, which the United States ratified. (From: The Health Effects of Cannabis and Cannabinoids: The Current State of Evidence and Recommendations for Research, the National Academy of Sciences)

This is the "Catch-22" or double blind created by the lawyers, and Congressmen, who wrote the Controlled Substances Act. They effectively took the power to make any laws related to marijuana away from future Congresses, and the American people, and placed these decisions into the hands of two appointed bureaucrats, and the United Nations. If the cure for cancer is found in the marijuana plant, American citizens continue to die of cancer because Congress created a law dependent on international treaties, instead of science, discovery, and alieving the suffering of their fellow man.

---

[13] http://www.cbc.ca/news/politics/trudeau-legalizing-pot-global-treaties-1.3390745

SECTION #4
The Placement of Marijuana on
Schedule 1 Hinders Research

I t is almost unanimous among Medical institutions, and think-tanks, that Marijuana's status as a Schedule 1 substance hinders research, and places doctors in legal jeopardy who would prescribe this drug. From the American Medical Association Journal of Ethics, we read:

"There are several barriers to physicians' prescribing marijuana for medical use. Although it remains illegal under federal law and is classified as a schedule 1 drug under the Controlled Substances Act (CSA) [7], 23 states and the District of Columbia have decriminalized its use for medicinal purposes [8]. Discrepancies between federal and state medicinal marijuana laws have placed doctors—and patients—in a difficult situation: to provide their patients with medicinal marijuana, doctors must risk violating federal law and, potentially, the revocation of their Drug Enforcement Agency (DEA) licenses." (Physicians, Medical Marijuana, and the Law. AMA Journal of Ethics, September 2014, Volume 16, Number 9.[14])

The status of marijuana as a Schedule 1 drug puts Doctors in a bind. Even if a patient does not respond to treatment, and is dying of a disease, it is illegal for them to prescribe Cannabis under

[14] http://journalofethics.ama-assn.org/2014/09/hlaw1-1409.html

the Law. They all must be licensed through the Drug Enforcement Agency, in order to prescribe medications. Therefore, all the warnings critics voiced regarding the Controlled Substances Act have come true. The Controlled Substances Act is mainly a law enforcement measure, instead of treating this problem as a health issue.

Numerous think-tanks, and physicians unions, have called for Cannabis to be rescheduled, including:

American Society of Regional Anesthesia and Pain Medicine

"The classification of marijuana as a Schedule 1 drug has hindered the generation of scientific evidence to evaluate the risks and benefits of marijuana use for medical purposes. Limitations imposed by federal agencies involved in approving clinical trials create challenges for investigators to conduct rigorous clinical research. Researchers must collaborate with three federal agencies in order to obtain study approval. Per the CSA, investigators are required to register with the DEA to obtain a site license, and submit an investigational new drug application (NDA) with the FDA. If a study is approved, the marijuana preparation must be obtained from the National Institute on Drug Abuse (NIDA).20 As a result of these barriers, there remains a dearth of high quality evidence available in the peer-reviewed literature regarding both the safety and efficacy of marijuana treatment." (American Society of Regional Anesthesia and Pain Medicine, Statement on Cannabis, Sept 30, 2016[15])

American College of Physicians
SUPPORTING RESEARCH INTO THE THERAPEUTIC ROLE OF MARIJUANA
A Position Paper of the American College of Physicians

"Currently, marijuana is a Schedule I controlled substance, meaning it has no medicinal value and high potential for abuse. An evaluation by several Department of Health and Human Services agencies, including the FDA and NIDA, concluded that no sound scientific studies supported medical

[15] https://www.asra.com/content/documents/full_asra_statement_on_cannabis.pdf

use of marijuana for treatment in the United States (39). This conflicts with a review by the IOM, which declared that "for patients such as those with AIDS or who are undergoing chemotherapy and who suffer simultaneously from severe pain, scientific studies support medical use of marijuana for treatment in the United States." The IOM also concluded that compared with other licit and illicit drugs, including alcohol, tobacco, and cocaine, "dependence among marijuana users is relatively rare and dependence appears to be less severe than dependence on other drugs." (40) A clear discord exists between the scientific community and federal legal and regulatory agencies over the medicinal value of marijuana, which impedes the expansion of research[16]."

American Nurses Association
Therapeutic Use of Marijuana and Related Cannabinoids

"It is the shared responsibility of professional nursing organizations to speak for nurses collectively in shaping health care and to promulgate change for the improvement of health and health care" (ANA, 2015, p. 36). Therefore, the ANA strongly supports:

• Scientific review of marijuana's status as a federal Schedule I controlled substance and relisting marijuana as a federal Schedule II controlled substance for purposes of facilitating research.

• Development of prescribing standards that includes indications for use, specific dose, route, expected effect and possible side effects, as well as indications for stopping a medication.

• Establishing evidence-based standards for the use of marijuana and related cannabinoids.

• Protection from criminal or civil penalties for patients using therapeutic marijuana and related cannabinoids as permitted under state laws.

[16]
https://www.acponline.org/acp_policy/policies/supporting_research_therapeutic_role_of_marijuana_2016.pdf

• Exemption from criminal prosecution, civil liability, or professional sanctioning, such as loss of licensure or credentialing, for health care practitioners who discuss treatment alternatives concerning marijuana or who prescribe, dispense or administer marijuana in accordance with professional standards and state laws.[17]"

Brooking's Institute

"Beyond interfering with the relationship between doctor and patient, the current policy stance toward medical marijuana and its research presents additional policy and practical challenges. Each day, patients, practitioners, hospitals, universities, and other public health professionals face tremendous questions about how federal drug policy can affect the practice of medicine and the daily operation of medical research and enterprise. The resulting legal gray area means that from day to day, state to state, practitioner to practitioner and even case to case the delivery of health care in the U.S. is interrupted and complicated by inconsistent and often contradictory policies. The irony of the issue is that it has very little to do with marijuana. This policy problem involves medical research and scientific freedom. This same conversation would be had if such barriers hindered the study of morphine or diazepam or Propofol or any other drug. Yet, of all the controlled substances that the federal government regulates, cannabis is treated in a unique manner in ways that specifically impede research." (Brookings Institute, Ending the U.S. Governments War on Marijuana Research, October 2015 [18])

These are merely a *few* well respected institutions that support rescheduling cannabis, so barriers to research can be removed. Many more have taken the same position. Our elected representatives are not just going against the will of the people— but also physicians, and medical institutions. The laws of the

[17] http://www.nursingworld.org/MainMenuCategories/Policy-Advocacy/Positions-and-Resolutions/ANAPositionStatements/Position-Statements-Alphabetically/Therapeutic-Use-of-Marijuana-and-Related-Cannabinoids.pdf

[18] https://www.brookings.edu/wp-content/uploads/2016/06/Ending-the-US-governments-war-on-medical-marijuana-research.pdf

United States hinder investigation; while numerous preclinical studies cry out for more research.

Recently, the United States Government relaxed some of the *regulations* regarding Marijuana, as a Schedule 1 substance. However, despite these reforms, many believe research will continue to be discouraged:

> "Medical research on marijuana probably won't get any easier, experts say, despite a new government policy aimed at boosting the supply of the drug for medical studies. That means the types of studies that are needed to address the safety and effectiveness of the drug as a medicine could still be a long way off. Marijuana's legal status as a "Schedule I" drug, which makes it an illegal drug on the federal level, "severely constrains the access and the number and type of people who can do research with cannabis," said Ryan Vandrey, an associate professor of psychiatry and behavioral sciences at The Johns Hopkins University School of Medicine who studies marijuana. "The unfortunate result of that is that we're now in a situation where you have literally millions of people using a drug for which we don't have established safety or efficacy data," Vandrey said." (Live Science, **New Medical Marijuana Policy Is a Catch-22, Researchers Say**
>
> By Rachael Rettner, Senior Writer | August 15, 2016[19])

About one year later, the prediction of these experts still holds true. According to a report in *Scientific American*, 25 applications "are still in review," but none have been granted approval[20].

While the United States government spends 4.9 billion of our tax dollars each year on cancer research, looking into *other* ways to cure cancer—it continues to ignore studies that point to a possible cure for cancer in cannabis. It continues to block, or impede research by refusing to reschedule cannabis. In fact, they have recently made laws *harder*, with additional controls placed on the concentrated oil of this plant…

---

[19] http://www.livescience.com/55765-new-medical-marijuana-policy-hinders-researchers.html

[20] https://www.scientificamerican.com/article/u-s-called-for-new-marijuana-research-bids-but-granted-no-approvals/

SECTION #5
The Continued Prohibition against Cannabis Oil

D espite many preclinical studies that demonstrate substances in marijuana can kill cancer cells, or slow the rate of their growth; despite news reports of miraculous cancer cures, and young children with epilepsy being successfully treated with Cannabis Oil; and despite many institutions of higher learning declaring that the placement of marijuana on "Schedule 1" is a hindrance to research— the United States government recently *tightened* the controls for this healing oil. In a press release about the placement of this concentrated oil in Schedule 1, we read:

"The United Nations Conventions on international drug control treats extracts from the cannabis plant somewhat differently than marihuana or tetrahydrocannabinols. The creation of a new drug code in the DEA regulations for marihuana extracts will allow for more appropriate accounting of such materials consistent with treaty provisions. The Single Convention on Narcotic Drugs, 1961 ("Single Convention") and the 1971 Convention on Psychotropic Substances ("Psychotropic Convention") provide for the international control of marihuana constituents. Many of the CSA's provisions were drafted to comply with these Conventions. The CSA includes schemes of drug scheduling and procedures for adding, removing, and transferring drugs among the schedules that are similar, in some ways, to those in the Single Convention. With respect to those drugs that are subject to control under the Single Convention, the CSA mandates that DEA control such drugs in a manner that will ensure the United States meets its obligations under the Single Convention. 21 U.S.C. 811(d)(1). Somewhat similar to the CSA, the Single Convention lists substances in four schedules. However, under the Single Convention, the drugs that are subject to the most stringent controls are in Schedule IV. Another difference between the CSA and the Single Convention is that, under the latter, a drug can be listed in more than one schedule. Cannabis and cannabis resin are listed in both Schedule IV and Schedule I of the Single Convention. Schedule I controls under the Single Convention include: Requirements for import and export authorization, licensing of manufacturers/distributors, record keeping requirements, a requirement for prescriptions for medical use, annual estimate of needs, quotas, annual statistical reporting, and a requirement that use be limited to medical and scientific purposes. Schedule II of the Single Convention is similar in controls to Schedule I with a few exceptions, and Schedule III is less restrictive. All substances listed in Schedule IV are also listed in Schedule I under the Single Convention in order to encompass the requirements mentioned above. In addition, as indicated, the Single Convention imposes certain heightened measures of control with respect to Schedule IV drugs. The placing of a drug into both Schedule I and Schedule IV, therefore imposes the most stringent controls under the Single Convention. Although cannabis and cannabis resin are listed in Schedules I and IV of the Single Convention, cannabis extracts are listed only in Schedule I.[21]" (From *Establishment of a New Drug Code for Marihuana Extract: A Rule by the Drug Enforcement Administration*)

This ruling is extremely troubling. First of all, they admit to the *real reason* they must control this drug. It is because they must keep "treaty provisions." It is not because of the health, and safety of the citizens of the United States. It is because the United States law has been written to comply with United Nations treaty protocols.

---

[21] Establishment of a New Drug Code for Marihuana Extract: A Rule by the Drug Enforcement Administration on 12/14/2016
https://www.federalregister.gov/documents/2016/12/14/2016-29941/establishment-of-a-new-drug-code-for-marihuana-extract

These protocols place Cannabis on a similar schedule, declaring it has no medicinal value.

It is also troubling because after all the news reports about this healing oil, the United States Government has *further criminalized it*. Testimonies of parents with children whose epileptic seizures were greatly reduced—or eliminated—by this oil have fallen on deaf ears. Although this oil does not "get you high," it has been placed in a higher schedule *only* because of the United Nations treaty.

Furthermore, the extraction of CBD oil from Hemp, or Flax, is also affected by this ruling. The government can shut down legitimate businesses that sell this oil. If they take these actions, they are hypocrites. From this article in the Washington Post, we find that some prescription drugs were approved *without* proper testing:

> "Pay attention, as I can't say this seriously enough. Last week, the FDA took a drug off the market, and the reasons should send shivers of fear down the backs of consumers, investors, generic drug companies – and the FDA. The FDA announced last week that the 300mg generic version of Wellbutrin XL manufactured by Impax Laboratories, and marketed by Teva Pharmaceuticals was being recalled because it did not work. And this wasn't just a problem with one batch – this is a problem that has been going on with this particular drug for four or five years, and the FDA did everything it could to ignore it. The FDA apparently approved this drug – and others like it – without testing it. The FDA just assumed if one dosage strength the drug companies submitted for approval works, then the other higher dosages work fine also. With this generic, American consumers became the FDA's guinea pigs to see if the FDA's assumption was right. It wasn't." (The Washington Post, October 10, 2012)

Many prescription drugs were not thoroughly tested, before being approved. In this instance, the green light was given to physicians by the government to prescribe this medication. Cannabis oil, on the other hand, is frequently given to patients who are *dying*. If someone is dying from an incurable cancer, what right does our government have to withhold this oil from them, leaving them with no other hope?

A medication or substance that could potentially cure incurable cancers should not be withheld from *anyone*. If people are dying, it is *wrong* to throw them in jail for treating their illness with a herb that is part of nature, that God created. If our elected representatives ignore the cry of the sick, and dying—and refuse to investigate this issue only to keep "international treaties[22]"— this is *callous*.

---

[22] The Controlled Substance Act

SECTION #6
The Endocannabinoid System

Research was partly funded in the late 1980's by the National Institute of Drug Abuse, to discover "receptors" in the human body for cannabis, similar to opiate receptors. These studies attempted to prove that marijuana was as addictive as opium. Instead, a vital signaling system in the human body was discovered. It was named the "endocannabinoid system" after cannabis, because marijuana acts as a "key" to "unlock," or affect these receptors. Although this is a vital system in the human body, many medical universities still do not teach about it in their classes.

The Endocannabinoid system explains how cannabis can treat many different diseases. Research was later funded to create synthetic analogs, that would affect the human body similar to marijuana—also "turning on" the cannabinoid receptors[23]. Some of these synthetic analogs were later sold in stores as "spice"—a legal substitute for marijuana. These substances almost turn people into "zombies," and are far more dangerous than cannabis.

Why was research funded to discover a substitute for marijuana? It only makes sense, if some people in our government *were aware* of the various medical uses for this plant, and attempted to find substitutes—that do not produce a "high." In this way, prescription medications could be created, and marijuana could remain illegal. The "spice" epidemic illustrates why the *natural* remedy is many times safer than a synthetic substitute.

---

[23] http://reason.com/blog/2012/08/01/how-the-national-institute-for-drug-abus

It also appears that our cannabinoid receptors affect the way our body responds to cancer. A recent study demonstrated that a *loss* of cannabinoid receptors can lead to colon cancer:

> "Two recent studies have shown that loss of CB1 led to an increase in carcinogenesis in colon cancer[169] and enhanced endocannabinoid tone prevented colon cancer,[170] thus pointing to a suppression of colon carcinogenesis by the ECS and CB1 receptor. Moreover, the CB2 receptor has been suggested to exert beneficial regulatory effects in the gut, such as attenuation of inflammation and probably colon cancer." (Cannabinoid receptor ligands as potential anticancer agents – high hopes for new therapies? Susanne Oescha and Jurg Gertsch.
>
> Journal of Pharmacy and Pharmacology, January 24, 2009[24])

It is *possible* that people with a deficiency in their cannabinoid receptors are more susceptible to cancer. Also, activating these receptors possibly explains how cannabinoids such as THC, THC-a, and CBD kill cancer cells. Conversely, activating these receptors through indigenous cannabinoids—such as anandamide—possibly explains the phenomenon of spontaneous remission. A few people might have extremely strong CB receptors, and produce cannabinoids naturally that fight the cancer. Furthermore, some people lack the digestive enzymes[25] to digest THC. This could be another reason some people have not responded to this treatment.

These subjective explanations should have either been proven—or disproved—*years* ago. It is possible everyone has receptors that activate at different levels. This would mean the same dosage of cannabis oil would not be the same for everyone, or even work for everyone. But again, only human trials can absolutely prove or disprove these possibilities—which should have been performed *decades ago*. Since the 1970's, research with *human subjects* into this possible cancer cure has been non-existent, because U. S. law has been written to comply with a treaty of the United Nations, and those in charge use regulations to halt investigation.

[24]http://theroc.us/images/Cannabinoid%20receptor%20ligands%20as%20potential%20anticancer%20agents%20%E2%80%93%20high%20hopes%20for%20new%20therapies.pdf

[25] Cytochrome P450 enzymes involved in the metabolism of tetrahydrocannabinols and cannabinol by human hepatic microsomes.
https://www.ncbi.nlm.nih.gov/pubmed/17303175

SECTION #7
Cannabis and Palliative Care

Research released in 1977 by the National Institute of Drug Abuse (quoted in section 2 of this book,) acknowledged that Cannabis is an effective pain killer. For this reason, Cannabis should be used in palliative care—instead of opiates—which cause constipation, extreme exhaustion, and nausea. Cannabis kills the pain *without* these side effects. In the American Journal of Hospice & Palliative Care, we read:

Cannabis in palliative medicine: improving care and reducing opioid-related morbidity.
"Opioids may produce significant morbidity. Cannabis is a safer alternative with broad applicability for palliative care. Yet the Drug Enforcement Agency (DEA) classifies cannabis as Schedule I (dangerous, without medical uses)...As palliative medicine grows, so does the need to reclassify cannabis. This article provides an evidence-based overview and comparison of cannabis and opioids. Using this foundation, an argument is made for reclassifying cannabis in the context of improving palliative care and reducing opioid-related morbidity." (The American Journal of Hospice & Palliative Care August 28, 2011[26])

This abstract states that Cannabis is a better choice in palliative care, because it reduces "opioid-related *morbidity*."

---

[26] https://www.ncbi.nlm.nih.gov/pubmed/21444324

Opiates are known to kill the patient quicker—and in 2002, we began to discover *why*. Drugs such as Morphine, Oxycontin, and similar pain killers, actually *spread cancer quicker*. We read this is Medical News Today:

> "New research from the US adds weight to the growing body of evidence that opiate-based painkillers like morphine, which has been used to treat postoperative and chronic cancer pain for two hundred years, encourage cancer cells to grow and spread. If confirmed with clinical studies, these findings could change the type of anasthetics given to cancer patients during surgery and the type of painkillers they use afterwards.
> Two new studies, presented last week at the "Molecular Targets and Cancer Therapeutics" meeting in Boston, Massachusetts, held by the American Association for Cancer Research, the National Cancer Institute, and the European Organization for Research and Treatment of Cancer, showed how shielding lung cancer cells from opiates reduced cell proliferation, invasion and migration in cell cultures and in mice. The studies were the work of Dr Patrick A Singleton, principal author of both studies and assistant professor of medicine at the University of Chicago Medical Center, and colleagues.
> The idea that opiates may play a role in cancer spread and recurrence has been gaining ground since 2002 when a palliative care trial showed that patients given spinal rather than systemic pain relief lived longer, the researchers told the press." (Opiate Painkillers May Encourage Spread Of Cancer. Medical News Today, Written by Catharine Paddock PhD, November 3, 2009[27])

This article states that the first studies revealed opiates spread cancer in *2002*. This was 25 years ago. During the past 25 years, how many cancer doctors continued to prescribe opiates to their patients? If they did, then logically, either one of two things are taking place. Either (a) this doctor has not kept up with the most recent studies or (b) this doctor knows this, and out of "compassion" is killing their patient *quicker*. This second choice might be okay, if the doctor *told* their patient: "I'm going to give you an opiate for the pain. I just want you to know, it will spread your cancer quicker." However, if the physician *knows* an opiate will

[27] http://www.medicalnewstoday.com/articles/171900.php

spread cancer quicker, but prescribes it to their patient anyway—*without telling them*—this is similar to manslaughter.

A doctor is not a "god," who decides who lives or dies. The patient has a right to know all risks of *any medication* the physician prescribes. The doctor might feel it is compassionate to kill a cancer patient quicker, but if the cancer spreads *quicker*, it would logically cause even *more* pain, and therefore, *more* opiates would be needed. This sets the patient on a "downhill spiral." Marijuana would be a better, *safer* choice. However, because of current law, physicians risk losing their licence to practice, if they prescribe[28] marijuana for the pain (or Cannabis Oil for the cancer itself.) This is true, even if traditional therapies (such as radiation or chemotherapy,) were pursued, and the patient did *not* respond, and has no other hope.

It has been known since NIDA's 1977 research monograph that cannabis has pain killing properties. For *four decades*, doctors have only had opiates—such as morphine—at their disposal for palliative care. You can thank the United States government, and the placement of Cannabis on Schedule 1, for limiting these physicians. It is possible the concentrated oil of this plant could slow the rate of cancer growth, or put it into remission, but Uncle Sam has stood in the way of *absolutely proving* any of this, by not funding any human clinical trials on cannabis as a cancer cure. Marijuana as a cancer cure might still be debatable; but not as a safer pain killer. It can kill the pain, without killing the patient—*as opiates do*.

Another serious condition physicians face in palliative care is Alzheimer's Disease. Despite the urban legend that marijuana causes "brain damage," the reality is actually *the opposite*. Marijuana helps treat—and reverse—neurodegeneration:

"Could medical marijuana treat Alzheimer's patients? One recent study found THC, the psychoactive ingredient in cannabis, stimulates the removal of toxic plaque in the brain, a common feature of the disease. Furthermore, the researchers discovered it blocks inflammation, which damages neurons in the brain. "It is reasonable to conclude that there is a therapeutic potential of cannabinoids for the treatment of Alzheimer's disease," wrote David Schubert, senior researcher and a professor at Salk Institute for

---

[28] In medical marijuana States, it is "recommended," *not* prescribed.

Biological Studies." (CNN, Medical marijuana has potential as Alzheimer's treatment, study says. By Susan Scutti, July, 25, 2016[29])

This is merely one recent study. Two years previously, in the Journal of Alzheimer's Disease, an article titled "The potential therapeutic effects of THC on Alzheimer's disease," we read:

"These sets of data strongly suggest that THC could be a potential therapeutic treatment option for Alzheimer's disease through multiple functions and pathways[30]."

These studies appear to present data that are revolutionary. The disease that ravaged Ronald Reagan, and so many other people, might *finally* have a cure. The problem is, the United States Government has known about this treatment *for years*, and has done nothing about it. In 2003, the government patented substances in cannabis to be used as a *neuroprotectant*:

United States Patent
6,630,507
Hampson, et al. October 7, 2003
Cannabinoids as antioxidants and neuroprotectants

Abstract
Cannabinoids have been found to have antioxidant properties, unrelated to NMDA receptor antagonism. This new found property makes cannabinoids useful in the treatment and prophylaxis of wide variety of oxidation associated diseases, such as ischemic, age-related, inflammatory and autoimmune diseases. The cannabinoids are found to have particular application as neuroprotectants, for example in limiting neurological damage following ischemic insults, such as stroke and trauma, or in the treatment of neurodegenerative diseases, such as Alzheimer's disease, Parkinson's disease and HIV dementia. Nonpsychoactive cannabinoids, such as cannabidiol, are particularly advantageous to use because they avoid toxicity that is encountered with psychoactive

---

[29] http://www.cnn.com/2016/07/25/health/alzheimers-medical-marijuana/
[30] https://www.ncbi.nlm.nih.gov/pubmed/25024327

cannabinoids at high doses useful in the method of the present invention[31].

The fact that the United States government obtained a patent for substances in Cannabis to treat neurodegenerative diseases—including Alzheimer's—is another *admission* of Marijuana's medicinal properties, proving that its placement on Schedule 1 is *a lie*. However, another fact about this patent is *extremely* troubling. *Fifteen years* have passed since the U.S. government was granted this patent. What has been done with it?

Where are the human subjects? Have studies been financed, to treat Alzheimer's patients of this illness? Not in the United States. In 2016, a small trial of human subjects in Israel was performed, with promising results[32]. This was almost 15 years after this patent was filed. If subsequent studies performed prove that substances in marijuana can treat Alzheimer's, this means your government did nothing with this patent for 15 years, while many of our mothers, fathers, and grandparents, *suffered in confusion, and died*.

[31] http://patft.uspto.gov/netacgi/nph-Parser?Sect1=PTO1&Sect2=HITOFF&d=PALL&p=1&u=%2Fnetahtml%2FPTO%2Fsrchnum.htm&r=1&f=G&l=50&s1=6630507.PN.&OS=PN%2F6630507&RS=PN%2F6630507

[32] http://www.jpost.com/Business-and-Innovation/Health-and-Science/Cannabis-may-offer-cure-for-dementia-study-finds-490233

SECTION #8
Does Marijuana Lead to Other Drugs?

Marijuana has been called a "gateway drug" by its critics. Some studies disagree, and have concluded instead that *alcohol* is actually the "gateway drug":

"A team of researchers from Texas A&M and the University of Florida examined data from 2,800 U.S. 12th graders interviewed for the Monitoring the Future study, an annual federal survey of teen drug use. They wanted to establish which substances teens typically used first. They give away their findings in the title of their paper: "Prioritizing Alcohol Prevention: Establishing Alcohol as the Gateway Drug and Linking Age of First Drink With Illicit Drug Use." They found that "the vast majority of respondents reported using alcohol prior to either tobacco or marijuana initiation." Not only that, but of those three main substances -- alcohol, tobacco and marijuana -- kids were the least likely to start using pot before the others." (The Washington Post. The Real 'Gateway Drug' is 100% legal. By Christopher Ingraham, January 6, 2016[33])

These researchers concluded that children were more likely to use alcohol before all these other substances. This makes sense, because children want to emulate adults, and prove their own adulthood. If they witness the adults use alcohol, alcohol will

---

[33] https://www.washingtonpost.com/news/wonk/wp/2016/01/06/the-real-gateway-drug-thats-everywhere-and-legal/?utm_term=.7e7d5c37bdcd

be the drug of "initiation." After this, they have crossed a line, and then breaking the *next* rule—and trying the *next* substance—is easier.

Many believe marijuana is a "gateway drug" because they believe it *does something to the brain*, that makes a person want to try *other* drugs. People who believe this have never used cannabis, and are projecting their own fears on this issue. Instead, marijuana use *does* lead to other drugs, but for a different reason. Once this reason is understood, it is obvious the U.S. government is actually *contributing* to the drug problem by their prohibition against marijuana.

It is inarguable that marijuana is the second or third most widely used drug, certainly after alcohol, and likely after tobacco. Alcohol and tobacco can be purchased in a store. In the majority of States, marijuana cannot. So, if a person want's to buy cannabis, where can they go? To a *drug dealer*.

They purchase weed from the black market. After a while, they build a relationship with their drug dealer. Then suddenly, their drug dealer *diversifies*. He has *more* than weed, but also cocaine, or Oxycodone. At this point, the person buying marijuana is *exposed to other drugs*, and possibly his drug dealer pressures him to buy them.

This is the real reason marijuana leads to other drugs. It is because it is usually sold on the black market *next to other drugs*. Usually, no one on heroin began on heroin. They were first consumers of marijuana, and buying marijuana on the black market exposed them to this drug.

For this reason, the United States government is actually *contributing* to the drug epidemic. In Colorado, marijuana is sold in a store with *no other drugs sold next to it.* Therefore, purchasing Cannabis legally in Colorado does *not* lead to other drugs. The drug *dealer* however, sells *everything*. The prohibitionist laws of the United States and the United Nations send cannabis customers to the drug dealers, and *some of them* try harder drugs because of this fact.

It is fallacy to believe that using *legal* Cannabis contributes to opiate addiction in the United States. In fact, States that have recreational or medical marijuana have seen a *decline* in opiate deaths:

"But using state-level death certificate data from 1999 to 2010, my colleagues and I found that the annual rate of opioid overdose deaths decreased substantially — by 25 percent on average — following the passage of medical marijuana laws, compared to states that still had bans. Could medical marijuana be a safer alternative to opioids for chronic pain management? If so, it would potentially reduce harms from opioid medicines." (The New York Times, Overdoses Fell with Marijuana Legalization. Colleen Barry. April 26, 2016[34])

Opiate overdoses likely fell because if people could choose which pain killer to use, they usually preferred Cannabis. The laws of the United States however, make extremely dangerous pain killers *legal* to use—drugs made from opium, or synthetic opiate analogues. These drugs are basically "legal heroin," and they *kill*. Cannabis does not. So, a medicine the Federal Government has approved for the treatment of pain *kills*, but people are locked up for using an herb for their pain *that kills no one*. Once again, it becomes apparent these laws against cannabis are indirectly killing people.

The same is true regarding alcohol use, and Cannabis law. Alcohol kills 60,000 people each year—and 20,000 of these are *overdose* deaths. Comparatively, there were 21,000 opiate overdose deaths in 2016. The opioid addiction problem is called a "crisis" for this reason—yet alcohol kills almost as many people.

Because the Federal Government has made a substance that kills legal, but a substance that kills no one illegal, the Government is partially to blame for these deaths. No matter how self-righteous a person feels regarding their own temperance, *a portion of the population* will always seek intoxication. The question is, will they have the ability to choose the *safer intoxicant*, or the more dangerous one?

Alcohol is far more debilitating than marijuana. Alcohol lowers inhibitions, With alcohol, it is easier to make bad choices. Unlike marijuana, people can get so drunk they do not know where they are. This fact makes marijuana far safer for drivers. Certainly, it is better not to drive intoxicated on either substance. However, anyone who has experienced *both* drugs knows that *alcohol is a harder drug*, incapacitating far more than marijuana.

[34] http://www.nytimes.com/roomfordebate/2016/04/26/is-marijuana-a-gateway-drug/overdoses-fell-with-medical-marijuana-legalization

Therefore, the marijuana laws passed by the United States government have aggregated drunk driving deaths. Many people would be alive today, if drunk drivers had instead used an intoxicant that *impairs less.*

Furthermore, alcohol has been implicated as a cause of several cancers. From the National Cancer Institute, we read:

"Most people know that heavy alcohol drinking can cause health problems. But many people might not know that drinking alcohol can raise their cancer risk. In fact, alcohol use is thought to account for about 3% to 4% of all cancer deaths each year in the United States. Alcohol is a known cause of cancers of the:

Mouth
Throat (pharynx)
Voice box (larynx)
Esophagus
Liver
Colon and rectum
Breast

Alcohol may also increase the risk of cancer of the pancreas. For each of these cancers, the risk increases with the amount of alcohol consumed." (Alcohol Use and Cancer.

The American Cancer Society. Cancer.gov[35])

The National Cancer Institute acknowledges that alcohol use can *increase* cancer risk, and at the same time, reports on their site that marijuana has anti-cancer, and anti-tumor effects. Of these two intoxicants, our government makes the intoxicant available that *increases* cancer risk, but it keeps the intoxicant illegal that could *reduce* cancer risk. Therefore, this is another government action that indirectly kills its citizens, and adds costs to our health care system.

---

[35] https://www.cancer.org/cancer/cancer-causes/diet-physical-activity/alcohol-use-and-cancer.html

SECTION #9
Marijuana and Stroke Risk

One objection that anti-Marijuana activists have recently raised is that Cannabis use is connected to a stroke risk. From CBS News, we read:

"New research analyzing millions of U.S. medical records suggests that marijuana use raises an adult's risk of stroke and heart failure. The study couldn't prove cause-and-effect, but the researchers said they tried to account for other heart risk factors. "Even when we corrected for known risk factors, we still found a higher rate of both stroke and heart failure in these patients," explained lead researcher Dr. Aditi Kalla, a cardiologist at Einstein Medical Center in Philadelphia." (From: Study Links Pot Use to Higher Risk for Stroke, Heart Failure. By Robert Preidt, March 10, 2017[36])

This press release made the headlines. However, the story published on *Motley Fool* rightly admits that this study—based on hospital visits—is flawed:

"Now, it's important to note that researchers were unable to prove that marijuana is the cause of the increase in stroke and heart attack risk. At this point their findings are merely correlative and worthy of additional research. For instance, researchers aren't able to determine the frequency of use for

[36] http://www.cbsnews.com/news/pot-marijuana-risk-stroke-heart-failure/

these 316,000 patients, the amount of use, or the delivery mechanism (smoking or ingestion). What's more, discharged patients may not be representative of the population." (Marijuana May Not Be as Safe as Proponents Claim, New Study Shows. Are pot users at an increased risk for stroke or heart attack? By Sean Williams. Mar 18, 2017[37])

This study conflicts with previous research. Instead of *constricting* blood vessels, studies have demonstrated that anandamide (an indigenous cannabinoid, which acts on the CB1 receptor in the same manner as THC) *reduces* blood pressure, by *opening* blood vessels:

Coronary vasodilator effects of endogenous cannabinoids in vasopressin-preconstricted unpaced rat isolated hearts
Journal of Cardiovascular Pharmacology
Sept 2005
Wagner JA, Abesser M, Karcher J, Laser M, Kunos G
Department of Internal Medicine I, Center of Cardiovascular Medicine, University of Würzburg, Würzburg, Germany.
"Delta-THC (10-100 nmol), the major psychoactive ingredient of cannabis, strongly decreased CF [coronary flow] and LVSP [left ventricular systolic pressure]. The CB2 receptor agonist JWH-133 (10-100 nmol) elicited vasodilator and positive inotropic effects only at higher doses. ...We conclude that in the rat isolated heart with reestablished vasoconstrictor tone, cannabinoids including anandamide elicit coronary vasodilation and a secondary increase in contractility via CB1 receptors and potassium channels[38]."

This is merely *one* study that confirms THC, and anandamide, are *vasodilators*. Vasodilators *protect* against a stroke. However, merely smoking, vaporizing, or ingesting marijuana a few times a month would not provide this kind of protection. Many people might have also eaten sushi a few times a month. That does not mean that eating sushi caused a stroke, any more than using marijuana infrequently.

---

[37] https://www.fool.com/investing/2017/03/18/marijuana-may-not-be-as-safe-as-proponents-claim-n.aspx

[38] https://www.ncbi.nlm.nih.gov/pubmed/16116341

Alcohol use however, is a different story. Studies have found that alcohol use in midlife (age 50 and above) raises the risk of stoke by 34%:

> "Too much alcohol in middle age can increase your stroke risk as much as high blood pressure or diabetes, a new study suggests. People who average more than two drinks a day have a 34 percent higher risk of stroke compared to those whose daily average amounts to less than half a drink, according to findings published Jan. 29 in the journal Stroke." (Too Much Alcohol at Midlife Raises Stroke Risk. The danger zone: more than 2 drinks daily. Web MD, Health Daily News, Jan 29, 2015[39])

When considering prohibition, our government is inconsistent. Any government official, or healthcare professional, who is shocked at the report that marijuana *might* raise stroke risk by 24%—and uses this report to discourage cannabis legalization— is either *ignorant* of studies linking alcohol to stroke risk, or is a hypocritical apologist for the anti-marijuana movement. The stroke risk associated with alcohol use is much *higher*.

---

[39] http://www.webmd.com/stroke/news/20150129/too-much-alcohol-at-midlife-raises-stroke-risk-study-finds

SECTION #10
Marijuana and Schizophrenia

A news story hit the wires early this year, that appears to link marijuana use with schizophrenia. NBC reported it as follows:

"Marijuana can help ease chronic pain but it can also raise the risk of severe mental illness, including schizophrenia, a comprehensive new report found. A team of top experts looked at all the studies that have been done on the use of cannabis — marijuana and products made from marijuana — and its impact on health. They can debunk some beliefs and raise a few warnings, but for the most part the committee appointed by the National Academies of Science, Engineering and Medicine said more study is needed." (NBC News, Marijuana Users Risk Schizophrenia, But the Drug Helps Pain. by Maggie Fox Jan 12, 2017[40])

Ever since this report was released from the National Academy of Sciences, dozens of articles have appeared, linking cannabis use to schizophrenia. Despite commentary in this report that interprets data in this manner, it also reveals the real reason marijuana use is linked to Schizophrenia. We read:

---

[40] http://www.nbcnews.com/health/health-news/report-marijuana-users-risk-schizophrenia-drug-helps-pain-n706196

"There is substantial evidence of a statistical association between cannabis use and: The development of schizophrenia or other psychoses, with the highest risk among frequent users."

In these words, we discover that these researchers simply acknowledged what has been known for a long time. There is a *statistical association* between cannabis use and schizophrenia. This means schizophrenics use marijuana at a *higher rate* than the rest of the population. We should ask the question however... "*why*?"

If marijuana *causes* schizophrenia symptoms, why do schizophrenics use it *more*? Symptoms of schizophrenia are debilitating. No one likes confusion. No one likes to hear voices, or live in constant fear, and paranoia. It appears to me, that schizophrenics might try marijuana *once*, and then be afraid of it for the rest of their lives—if it *causes* schizophrenic symptoms.

The National Academy of Sciences analyzed several studies that noted this statistical relationship. Yet, if you read the "fine print," *all* of these studies raise the possibility that schizophrenics are actually using marijuana at a higher rate to *treat their disease*. This observation has been reported in the Psychiatry Advisor:

"The connection between cannabis use and psychiatric disorders, particularly schizophrenia, is supported by a large body of research, but the debate continues as to whether one has a more causative effect than the other. A common argument against marijuana legalization, for example, is that the drug is associated with increased psychosis risk. Though causation has not been established, these criticisms imply that cannabis use results in psychosis. It is unclear whether that is the case or if people with psychotic disorders are engaging in a form of self-medication....Given the increased rates of cannabis use among people with schizophrenia, along with the role of the endocannabinoid system in the pathophysiology of the disease, some experts have begun investigating whether some cannabinoids could help manage some of the symptoms of schizophrenia." (Psychiatry Advisor, Cannabis and Schizophrenia: Trigger or Treatment? February 23, 2015[41])

The connection between increased cannabis use among schizophrenics is only logically explained if they are self medicating. For the same reason, there is also a higher incidence of alcohol use among schizophrenics:

"Evidence suggests that there are elevated rates of alcohol-use disorders (AUDs) at each stage of schizophrenia. Although the literature examining the clinical implications of alcohol at the early stages of schizophrenia are rather sparse, findings from numerous studies suggest that comorbid AUDs in individuals with schizophrenia exacerbate psychopathology, undermine medication compliance, add to cognitive dysfunction, impaired community functioning and physical health....For individuals with schizophrenia, the use of alcohol can become a common means to regulate or cope with a distressful affective state [27–30] as they tend to lack the necessary problem solving skills and strategies to successfully cope with stress." (Clinical implications of alcohol-use disorders in schizophrenia. Matthew J Smith, John G Csernansky)

Now, if I wanted dishonestly to create an argument for alcohol prohibition, I could correlate this evidence in the same manner as the researchers who pose that cannabis *causes* schizophrenia. I could say "there is a higher incidence of alcohol use among schizophrenics, therefore, alcohol use is *causing* schizophrenia." Yet, as this article states, the schizophrenics are likely using alcohol because they are in a "distressful state," and these people "undermine medication compliance." In these words, we discover the real reason schizophrenics use alcohol: *self medication*.

I have known people with this disease. It is *not* fun. Having delusions, and being paranoid all of the time, is something that a schizophrenic would *hate*. Why smoke marijuana if it exasperates these symptoms?

[41] http://www.psychiatryadvisor.com/schizophrenia-and-psychoses/cannabis-and-schizophrenia-trigger-or-treatment/article/399675/

As stated, the second most prevalent substance in marijuana is CBD, or Cannabidiol. Researchers have discovered that this substance in cannabis is as effective as prescription anti-psychotics:

A critical review of the antipsychotic effects of cannabidiol: 30 years of a translational investigation.

Current Pharmaceutical Design
2012

Zuardi AW, Crippa JA, Hallak JE, Bhattacharyya S, Atakan Z, Martin-Santos R, McGuire PK, Guimarães FS
Department of Neuroscience and Behavior, Faculty of Medicine, University of São Paulo and National Institute for Translational Medicine, Ribeirão Preto, SP-Brazil.

Abstract

$\Delta(9)$-tetrahydrocannabinol ($\Delta(9)$-THC) is the main compound of the Cannabis Sativa responsible for most of the effects of the plant. Another major constituent is cannabidiol (CBD), formerly regarded to be devoid of pharmacological activity. However, laboratory rodents and human studies have shown that this cannabinoid is able to prevent psychotic-like symptoms induced by high doses of $\Delta(9)$- THC. Subsequent studies have demonstrated that CBD has antipsychotic effects as observed using animal models and in healthy volunteers. Thus, this article provides a critical review of the research evaluating antipsychotic potential of this cannabinoid. CBD appears to have pharmacological profile similar to that of atypical antipsychotic drugs as seem using behavioral and neurochemical techniques in animal models. Additionally, CBD prevented human experimental psychosis and was effective in open case reports and clinical trials in patients with schizophrenia with a remarkable safety profile. Moreover, fMRI results strongly suggest that the antipsychotic effects of CBD in relation to the psychotomimetic effects of $\Delta(9)$-THC involve the striatum and temporal cortex that have been traditionally associated with psychosis. Although the mechanisms of the antipsychotic properties are still not fully understood, we propose a hypothesis that could have a heuristic value to inspire new studies. These results support the idea that CBD may be a future therapeutic option in psychosis, in general and in schizophrenia, in particular[42]."

The drugs used for schizophrenia have terrible side effects. Schizophrenics, therefore, seek alternative methods of treatment. Since alcohol is legal in all 50 states, it is the easiest non-prescription drug schizophrenics can obtain. Cannabis is the second most prevalent substance. And, the study quoted above demonstrates that CBD (Cannabidiol) can *treat* schizophrenia as effectively as current medications, without the severe side effects.

---

[42] https://www.ncbi.nlm.nih.gov/pubmed/22716160

Since studies indicate that a substance in marijuana can treat schizophrenia, it is almost certain that schizophrenics use marijuana at a higher rate than the rest of the population because they are self-medicating their disease. CBD in Cannabis has less side effects than current schizophrenic medications. Furthermore, many violent acts have been committed by patients after *suddenly withdrawing* from anti-depressants, and anti-psychotics. Cannabis would be a safer alternative to these drugs.

The ability for researchers to develop safer medications from marijuana, to treat mental diseases, has been impeded by the regulations of current law.

SECTION #11
Research Skewed by Low Grade Cannabis

The National Academy of Sciences correctly states in their report that *more research is needed.* However, some of the abstracts in their analysis used *extremely low grade* marijuana, grown in Mississippi:

"But if you're a researcher looking to work with marijuana — to say, investigate how it impairs people, or how it could help people suffering from certain ailments—you don't have access to the weed that everyone else is using. Since the late 1960s the federal government has mandated that all marijuana used in research has to come through the federal government. To investigate the real-world effects of marijuana, however, researchers need a product that looks and feels like the real thing. And they're increasingly frustrated with government weed that is something else entirely. Don't take their word for it. The photo below shows a sample of federal marijuana distributed to Sue Sisley, a researcher who just embarked on a first-of-its-kind clinical trial to test the efficacy of medical marijuana for military veterans suffering from PTSD." (Washington Post, Government marijuana looks nothing like the real stuff. See for yourself. By Christopher Ingraham and Tauhid Chappell March 13, 2017[43])

---

[43]https://www.washingtonpost.com/news/wonk/wp/2017/03/13/government-marijuana-looks-nothing-like-the-real-stuff-see-for-yourself/?utm_term=.4f4b51e6aa8

The marijuana Dr. Sisley received from the government was extremely low potency marijuana—something called "dirt weed" on the street—merely *slightly* more potent as Hemp. Some Scientists believe that their research is being hindered *on purpose*, in order to keep marijuana illegal:

"The National Institute on Drug Abuse, a branch of the National Institutes of Health, administers the program and in late March granted Ole Miss a $68.7 million contract renewal, effectively upholding the university's distinction as America's legal weed supplier. In doing so, the government ended speculation that the feds might expand the program or move it elsewhere. As more and more states and cities move toward legalization or decriminalization of marijuana, interest in the Mississippi lab and the research conducted there has also grown, as has resentment at what critics decry as Mississippi's monopoly on growing legal pot. Specifically, scientists have become increasingly disgruntled about having to jump through countless regulatory hoops to procure Mississippi marijuana for their research. And because the federal government – namely the U.S. Drug Enforcement Agency – still classifies marijuana as a Schedule I narcotic, along with other powerful drugs like meth and heroin, the DEA also gets to sign off on research proposals. Critics of the process argue that because the DEA has a vested interest in keeping marijuana illegal, the agency gives preference to studies that are likely to highlight marijuana's harmful effects." (International Business Times. How A Mississippi Lab Taught Us Everything We Know About Marijuana, For Better Or Worse By R.L. Nave 04/22/15.[44])

Unless our government is ignorant of the potency of their marijuana strains, low grade marijuana has been grown on purpose to derail researchers, so they will not discover plant's medicinal effects. Sue Sisley is performing the first clinical trial to discover if marijuana can treat Post Traumatic Stress Disorder (PTSD), a terrible psychological condition suffered by our soldiers, many times leading to suicide.

---

[44] http://www.ibtimes.com/how-mississippi-lab-taught-us-everything-we-know-about-marijuana-better-or-worse-1890470

This low grade Cannabis was given as either a one-time attempt to derail Dr. Sisley's study—at the expense of our veterans—or it is given to all researchers, to *derail all Cannabis studies*. If the former, there was a complete disregard for our men and women in uniform. If the latter, there has been a complete disregard for *all* citizens, because *all* cannabis studies have been skewed by this low grade cannabis.

The use of this poor quality marijuana explains the existence of many conflicting studies. For instance, some studies purport that marijuana *raises* blood pressure, some that it *lowers* it. Since any substance smoked creates carbon monoxide, and other toxic gasses, inhaling these gasses can raise the blood pressure, and Cortisol levels. This is true *no matter what* is being smoked: cigarettes, herbs, or marijuana.

If the subjects in clinical trials had to smoke several joints to achieve a "buzz" in these studies, the frequency, and amount, of low grade marijuana smoked could cause several bad effects. Conversely, higher potency marijuana requires less plant material to be smoked, and thus less inhalation of these toxic gasses. The effect of ingested, or vaporized marijuana would be vastly different.

Ronald Reagan believed a flawed study, that appeared to prove marijuana caused brain damage. After the details of the study were released, everyone recognized its flaw. Researchers strapped gas masks to monkeys, and they were forced to smoke *dozens* of joints, one after another[45]. Of course they got brain damage—from carbon monoxide poisoning.

All these studies performed with the low grade Cannabis grown in Mississippi are possibly spurious, because more marijuana would be smoked, and the gasses inhaled when smoking a large amount of *any substance* has deleterious effects. Of course, the quality of the study would be affected by the quality of the drug used. The low grade marijuana grown in Mississippi for research could be an attempt to hide the benefits of Cannabis —including a possible cancer cure.

[45] http://www.upressonline.com/2016/09/opinion-cannabis-could-help-prevent-long-term-damage-from-concussions/

SECTION #12
Our Rights have been Violated

A natural right to treat our afflictions with a plant given to us by God, and nature, has been violated by a law created by Richard Nixon, and the 91st Congress. Furthermore, our first amendment rights have also been violated by this law.

In the United States Constitution, we read:

> Congress shall make no law respecting an establishment of religion, or prohibiting the free exercise thereof; or abridging the freedom of speech, or of the press, or the right of the people peaceably to assemble, and to petition the Government for a redress of grievances.

The first amendment states that Congress cannot make *any* law that "abridges" "the right of the people" "to petition the Government for a redress of grievances." Now, although a procedure exists in the Controlled Substances Act to petition the government regarding this issue, the "redress" of this grievance no longer exists with the Government of the United States. Instead, the Controlled Substance Act gives the United Nations precedence over the decisions of the Attorney General. Therefore, since Congress created a law that gives the power of "redress" to the U.N.—the ability to petition our own Government for a "redress" *has been abridged*.

The Controlled Substances Act, the U.N. Convention on Psychotropic Substances, and the United States Psychotropic

73

Substances Act, are all laws created by Congress that abridges our right to petition our Government about an issue regarding the treatment of our health. These laws take the ability to reschedule a medicinal substance away from the United States government, Congress, the Attorney General, and the American people—and places this power in the hands of the Secretary General of the United Nations, and the World Health Organization. Therefore, our first amendment rights have been violated. Congress has created a law that "abridged" the right of the people to petition their government, because the final decision for a "redress" of this grievance has been given to a different government body—the United Nations.

SECTION #13
Conclusions

Over 100 preclinical studies show promising results of substances in marijuana for a treatment of cancer— listed in the appendix of this book. Yet, there has not been one human trial in the United States to investigate these results. In my opinion, these studies—coupled with dozens of human testimonies—means this is likely true. However, what occurs in a rat or test tube might not take place in a human being. Furthermore, cannabinoids could work differently according to a person's genetic makeup. In other words, the dosage of cannabis oil, and its effectiveness, could vary according to an individuals "cannabinoid receptors."

This possibility should have been answered *decades* ago. The government has left cannabis-cancer research in limbo, because no studies have been performed on humans to confirm— or deny— this preclinical evidence. And, *if true*, how many could have been saved of cancer, since the first study was released in 1974? After all the preclinical evidence, why has there not been any funding for human clinical trials? Why have the people in our government made performing research in this issue *next to impossible*?

Every year, *thousands* die from these various cancers:

Bladder 16,870
Breast 40,610
Colon and Rectal 50,260
Endometrial 10,920
Kidney 14,400
Leukemia 24,500
Liver 28,920
Lung 155,870
Melanoma 9,730
Non-Hodgkin Lymphoma 20,140
Prostate 26,730
Thyroid 2,010

Total: 390,820

Consider the implications of current law. If human trials eventually prove that substances in Cannabis *can* cure cancer, the United States Government has done a great disservice to its people. The Controlled Substances Act has delayed the exploration of this cancer cure. About every 6 years, the government spends 4.9 billion of *your* tax dollars on cancer research[46]. This research looks into *other* possible treatments for cancer, usually with futility. Yet, numerous preclinical studies point to indigenous, synthetic, and phytocannabinoids (plant based) as a possible cancer cure. Yet, the Government is *not interested*. ZERO has been spent to investigate this issue.

Every year the Government drags its feet, 390,000 people suffer and die of cancer that possibly could be saved. These are real people who are suffering—men, women, and children. They could be *your* relatives, *your* parents, or *your* children. Anyone who has witnessed someone die of cancer, has been touched by the extreme agony of this disease. The preclinical evidence raises the possibility that their suffering could have been avoided.

We must fund research to find the truth. A doctor can truthfully say "there is *no evidence* that substances in marijuana cure cancer." However, these words are only *technically* true, because the Government will not fund any *human clinical trials*. Only if human trials are performed, can the truth be discovered.

---

[46] http://blogs.reuters.com/stories-id-like-to-see/2014/09/09/the-money-spent-in-fighting-cancer-and-alibabas-risk-factor/

In order to keep an international treaty, research has been derailed. It is possible 390,000 people die each year in America of cancer, because our drug laws have been written to be compliant with this treaty. The majority of our elected representatives are ignorant this issue. They are unaware about the numerous studies that reveal substances in marijuana can kill cancer cells.

After the first studies revealed this in 1970's, money should have *immediately* been invested into research. Instead, funds were allocated by Congress into *other* possible cancer cures. In the meantime, a legalistic snake of red tape continued to hinder researchers who would investigate this issue, because Marijuana has been declared to be a substance that has no medicinal value.

Deaths from Other Conditions

If substances in Cannabis can cure cancer, and research has been delayed by current law, the United States Government is partially culpable in 390,000 deaths each year. Furthermore, there are several deadly conditions Cannabis could possibly treat, according to literature released from the National Institute of Drug Abuse in 1977. As quoted in the second section of this book, the publication "Marihuana Research Findings: 1976" reveals that these conditions can be treated by Cannabis:

Bronchodilation
Anticonvulsant
Analgesia
Antidepressant
Treatment of Alcohol and Drug Dependence

The 1977 report also affirms that Cannabis has anti-tumor activity, an admission of anti-cancer effects. It also acknowledges marijuana as an anti-nausea medication, which would also save lives. The U.S. Government however, has developed a synthetic cannabinoid, Marinol, to be used for nausea. The government had to petition the United Nations to reschedule this substance. So, they have helped save some lives by *this* action.

It is possible that some of the lives lost in the five categories listed above could have been saved. Failure to invest in the development of new medications from Cannabis to treat these conditions possibly has resulted in the deaths of thousands of men, women, and children. Let's consider the deaths caused by each of these conditions:

1. Bronchodilation

Cannabis has the ability to open up air passages, and lungs. Therefore, it can treat asthma. Two years before NIDA's report, a study was completed that concluded that marijuana could treat asthma:

Effects of smoked marijuana in experimentally induced asthma.
American Review of Respiratory Disease
Tashkin DP, Shapiro BJ, Lee YE, Harper CE
September 1975.

Abstract:
"After experimental induction of acute bronchospasm in 8 subjects with clinically stable bronchial asthma, effects of 500 mg of smoked marijuana (2.0 per cent delta9-tetrahydrocannabinol) on specific airway conductance and thoracic gas volume were compared with those of 500 mg of smoked placebo marijuana (0.0 per cent delta9-tetrahydrocannabinol), 0.25 ml of aerosolized saline, and 0.25 ml of aerosolized isoproterenol (1,250 mug). Bronchospasm was induced on 4 separate occasions, by inhalation of methacholine and, on four other occasions, by exercise on a bicycle ergometer or treadmill. Methacholine and exercise caused average decreases in specific airway conductance of 40 to 55 per cent and 30 to 39 per cent, respectively, and average increases in thoracic gas volume of 35 to 43 per cent and 25 to 35 per cent, respectively. After methacholine-induced bronchospasm, placebo marijuana and saline inhalation produced minimal changes in specific airway conductance and thoracic gas volume, whereas 2.0 per cent marijuana and isoproterenol each caused a prompt correction of the bronchospasm and associated hyperinflation. After exercise-induced bronchospasm, placebo marijuana and saline were followed by gradual recovery during 30 to 60 min, whereas 2.0 per cent marijuana and isoproterenol caused an immediate reversal of exercise-induced asthma and hyperinflation[47]."

Another study reported similar results. In a 1973 article published in the New England Journal of Medicine, titled *"Single-Dose Effect of Marihuana Smoke—Bronchial Dynamics and Respiratory-Center Sensitivity in Normal Subjects"* we read:

"Normal volunteers with previous marihuana smoking experience inhaled the total smoke from 3.23 mg per kilogram of marihuana, using a bag-in-box technic.

---

[47] https://www.ncbi.nlm.nih.gov/pubmed/1099949

Randomly, nine received marihuana containing a high (2.6 per cent), and eight a low (1.0 per cent) concentration of delta-9 tetrahydrocannabinol. Physiologic variables were monitored before and for 20 minutes after smoking. In the high-dose group the heart rate increased 28 per cent. Concomitantly, airway resistance, measured in a body plethysmograph, fell 38 per cent; the functional residual capacity remained unchanged (± 50 ml) throughout, and specific airway conductance increased 44 per cent. Flow-volume loops showed a 45 per cent increase in flow rate at 25 per cent of vital capacity. The low-dose group showed no increase in heart rate but significant, if lesser changes, in airways dynamics. Carbon dioxide sensitivity, measured by rebreathing remained unchanged in both groups. Marihuana smoke, unlike cigarette smoke, causes bronchodilatation rather than bronchoconstriction and, unlike opiates, does not cause central respiratory depression[48]." (New England Journal of Medicine 288:985–989, 1973)

These subjects were given a very low dose of marijuana, which means they had to smoke *more* to achieve the same effect of *a few puffs* of higher potency Cannabis. Nevertheless, the ability to treat asthma with Cannabis was *noted in 1974*, and reported to Congress in 1977. Yet, Marijuana continued to be placed in the most restrictive Schedule, which made further studies into this issue *rare*.

The inability to treat asthma effectively results in 250,000 deaths each year. If cannabis can treat asthma, the United States government is partially to blame for these deaths. They had evidence, and did *nothing* about it. Furthermore, as many as 80 percent of these deaths might be caused by the asthma *medications:*

"Three common asthma inhalers containing the drugs salmeterol or formoterol may be causing four out of five U.S. asthma-related deaths per year and should be taken off the market, researchers from Cornell and Stanford universities have concluded after a search of medical literature." ("Common asthma inhalers cause up to 80 percent of asthma-

[48] New England Journal of Medicine 288: 985-989, 1973.
http://www.nejm.org/doi/full/10.1056/NEJM197305102881902

related deaths, Cornell and Stanford researchers assert. Cornell Chronicle. March 21, 2017. By Krishna Ramanujan[49])

The U.S. Government has known for *40 years* that substances in cannabis could treat asthma. Yet, they have refused to reschedule it, preventing research. Many of these 250,000 deaths were *children*, killed by the medication their government deemed to be safe. The ability to make a safer medication from cannabis for asthma has been continuously delayed because of current law.

2. Anticonvulsant
There are an estimated 50,000 deaths from epilepsy each year. Many take multiple medications, without any relief. The majority of people who die from epilepsy are those who have the most seizures. Cannabis oil has proven to relieve these seizures in some people (either THC-a oil, or CBD oil, depending on the type of epilepsy.) The prescription medications given for epilepsy can have severe side effects, and in some cases are debilitating.
The inability to create, and test, a drug from Cannabis to treat epilepsy has possibly resulted in thousands of deaths each year. The National Institute of Drug Abuse admitted that Cannabis could possibly treat this disease in 1977—and there was *no follow-up*.

3. Analgesia
Opiate pain killers—and other opiates—caused 21,000 deaths last year, and countless deaths since the 1970's, when NIDA's 1977 report was released. Because opiates are physically addicting, many begin with *prescription* pain killers, but end up on heroin. The U.S. Government knew in 1977 that cannabis is an effective pain killer, *without* the risk of overdose. Instead of rescheduling this drug, so it could be prescribed as a pain killer, they made opiates more readily available to the population, and are therefore partially to blame for the current opioid epidemic.

4. Antidepressant
Antidepressant overdoses are the second cause of deaths from all drug overdoses. No one has ever died from a Marijuana overdose, yet our government has approved many antidepressants that are dangerous, in many ways. Sudden withdrawal from these

[49] http://www.news.cornell.edu/stories/2006/06/common-asthma-inhaler-causing-deaths-researchers-assert

medications can cause delusions leading to violence, and some medications themselves can lead to suicide:

> "Antidepressants can raise the risk of suicide, the biggest ever review has found, as pharmaceutical companies were accused of failing to report side-effects and even deaths linked to the drugs. An analysis of 70 trials of the most common antidepressants - involving more than 18,000 people - found they doubled the risk of suicide and aggressive behaviour in under 18s. Although a similarly stark link was not seen in adults, the authors said misreporting of trial data could have led to a 'serious under-estimation of the harms.'" (Antidepressants can raise the risk of suicide, biggest ever review finds. The Telegraph By Sarah Knapton, Science Editor. January 27, 2016[50])

Many of these people who committed suicide were *teenagers*, and *young adults*. Our government has approved these drugs to treat depression, but research into a drug from cannabis to treat depression has not been performed since its antidepressant properties were recognized in NIDA's 1977 report. Since that time, countless people have taken these drugs, and many have ended their lives in suicide. Current law constrains research to create a drug made from cannabis for depression that has no psychoactive effects, and lacks the *dangerous* side effects of current medications.

5. Treatment of Alcohol and Drug Dependence

As stated, 20,000 people die each year from alcohol overdose. In the 1977 report to Congress, we read that marijuana could be used in the treatment of alcoholism, and drug dependence. Instead, many in government embraced a "gateway drug" theory, erroneously believing that cannabis does "something to the brain" that makes people crave *other* drugs. In NIDA's report, we discover the *opposite*. And, the fact that opiate deaths have *fallen* in every State that has approved medical marijuana laws, prove NIDA's observations were correct. This was a rare time in their history, when truth prevailed over government propaganda.

---

[50] http://www.telegraph.co.uk/science/2016/03/14/antidepressants-can-raise-the-risk-of-suicide-biggest-ever-revie/

NIDA also reported in 1977 that Cannabis has *anti-tumor* effects. Despite this report, the United States Government has continued to place marijuana in the strictest category, a declaration of no medicinal value. This decision has led to a man's death, who suffered from grape-fruit sized tumors protruding throughout his body. Cannabis oil reduced the size of these tumors, and kept this man alive. Before he was sentenced, he stated that a conviction would lead to his death:

"A dying man who claims he grew marijuana to treat a painful cancer faces a possible prison sentence after a conviction on drug charges Wednesday — a prospect he views as a "death sentence. Scott County jurors delivered a guilty verdict on four felony drug charges facing Benton Mackenzie, 48, whose wife and son were also convicted alongside him. Mackenzie says he used the plants to extract cannabis oil to treat a painful grapefruit-sized tumor on his buttock caused by angiosarcoma, a rare, aggressive cancer." (USA Today, Cancer patient says pot conviction a 'death sentence' July 10, 2014[51])

Since neither the United States Government, or the State of Iowa, recognized the medicinal properties of marijuana, the judge would not allow a medical necessity defense. It was not long however, until this man died of his disease while on probation, unable to use marijuana:

"Even as he faced his final moments, Benton Mackenzie's first thoughts were of his wife and son and their future. The 49-year-old terminal cancer patient who fought Scott County authorities over his efforts to grow marijuana for his own medicinal use died early Monday at home....As Mackenzie stood trial, his health deteriorated. The baggy sweatpants he wore masked huge cancerous tumors covering his rear and right leg, a symptom of the angiosarcoma he was diagnosed with in 2011. He was rushed to an emergency room in the middle of his trial for a blood transfusion. Jurors were not allowed to hear any testimony about his health and convicted him along with Loretta for conspiring to grow marijuana. Their

[51] http://www.usatoday.com/story/news/nation/2014/07/10/cancer-patient-calls-marijuana-conviction-death-sentence/12468445/

son, Cody, was convicted of drug possession. They all were sentenced to probation in September, and as his rare cancer progressed into the final stages, Benton Mackenzie spent the remaining months of 2014 mostly confined to a hospice bed at his parents' basement apartment in Long Grove." (Family of Benton Mackenzie mourns his death. The Quad City Times. By Brian Wellner. Jan 13, 2015)

While on probation, he was not allowed to use Cannabis oil, *so he died.* He died *suffering,* of huge tumors growing out of his body. Consider this news report, in light of NIDA's report in 1977. Back then—four decades ago—our government knew that marijuana had anti-tumor effects. However, *instead* of funding research, the government *continued prohibition.* This prohibition took away the right of this man to treat his disease, and he died because of it.

Yet, this is merely *one* man who suffered and died. The list of deaths caused by these laws could be astronomical. 390,000 Cancer deaths; 20,000 Alcohol overdose deaths; 250,000 Asthma deaths; 21,000 opiate deaths, and 50,000 death from seizures. This means that each year, it is possible that 731,000 die indirectly due to Cannabis prohibition.

"Good People"

The reasons people in our government want to continue cannabis prohibition are numerous, and to speculate that it is one "conspiracy" is incorrect. Certainly, there is evidence that some politicians take money from the liquor, or pharmaceutical industry to keep marijuana illegal. However, the majority of these anti-marijuana opinions arise from complete ignorance of this drug. For instance, Attorney General Jeff Sessions once said:

"Good people don't smoke marijuana."

He is completely off base. Instead, *good people would not hold back a cancer cure from the public. Good people would not let people suffer, by holding back a plant that can ease their suffering. Good people would not hold back a treatment for asthma attacks, or seizures.* That is exactly what our elected representatives are guilty of, if they *know about this promising research*, and *do nothing about it.*

If the United States finally tests the substances in cannabis on human subjects, and these cannabinoids do *not* heal cancer, then the U.S. Government will exonerate itself. However, if this is proven to be true—and the U.S. continues to put off human testing—Uncle Sam will eventually be caught with his "pants down." The cat will be "let out of the bag." *Another country* will eventually perform this research. It might be Israel, the United Kingdom, France, or Australia. If any of these nations perform these human clinical trials *with success*, it will then be *obvious to everyone* that United States cannabis prohibition has contributed to the deaths of thousands its citizens.

Why We Should Look Here for a Cure *First*

Every year, numerous treatments for cancer are tested, and almost none of them had over 100 preclinical studies to warrant further investigation. Cannabis *does*, yet there has been no follow up.

There is a good reason scientists, and researchers should investigate Cannabis as a cancer treatment: *the endocannabinoid system*. Researchers are discovering that turning these receptors "on" fights cancer, but turning them "off" accelerates cancer growth. Since this is a vital system in the human body, attempting to cure cancer with chemotherapeutic agents that work *outside* of this system could be in vain. Substances in marijuana directly influence this system, which is why researchers should look here *first*.

Because a cure for cancer might lie in the concentrated oil of this plant, we must rise up against the prohibition of this plant. If the United Nations does not reschedule Cannabis, the United States must *pull out* of the U.N. Convention on Psychotropic Substances. The Controlled Substances Act must be amended, or repealed, to allow Cannabis to be rescheduled without U.N. interference. Government funding must be invested in Cannabis-Cancer research. And, while we wait on the results of these much needed human clinical trials, everyone should have access to this oil, especially people with *no treatment options*. It is wrong for the United States to withhold it from its citizens, which could prove to be their only chance for life.

OVER 100
CANNABIS-CANCER STUDIES
1974-2016

1974

Antineoplastic Activity of Cannabinoids.
Journal of the National Cancer Institute
Munson AE, Harris LS, Friedman MA, Dewey WL, Carchman RA.

Abstract
Lewis lung adenocarcinoma growth was retarded by the oral administration of delta9-tetrahydrocannabinol (delta9-THC), delta8-tetrahydrocannabinol (delta8-THC), and cannabinol (CBN), but not cannabidiol (CBD). Animals treated for 10 consecutive days with delta9-THC, beginning the day after tumor implantation, demonstrated a dose-dependent action of retarded tumor growth. Mice treated for 20 consecutive days with delta8-THC and CBN had reduced primary tumor size. CBD showed no inhibitory effect on tumor growth at 14, 21, or 28 days. Delta9-THC, delta8-THC, and CBN increased the mean survival time (36% at 100 mg/kg, 25% at 200 mg/kg, and 27% at 50 mg/kg, respectively), whereas CBD did not. Delta9-THC administered orally daily until death in doses of 50, 100, or 200 mg/kg did not increase the life-spans of (C57BL/6 times DBA/2)F1 (BDF1) mice hosting the L1210 murine leukemia. However, delta9-THC administered daily for 10 days significantly inhibited Friend leukemia virus-induced splenomegaly by 71% at 200 mg/kg as compared to 90.2% for actinomycin D. Experiments with bone marrow and isolated Lewis lung cells incubated in vitro with delta9-THC and delta8-THC showed a dose-dependent $(10(-4)-10(-7))$ inhibition (80-20%, respectively) of tritiated thymidine and 14C-uridine uptake into these cells. CBD was active only in high concentrations $(10(-4))$.

PubMed Link: https://www.ncbi.nlm.nih.gov/pubmed/1159836

Retardation of Tumor Growth by Delta-9-tetrahydrocanabinol
The Pharmacologist
Munson AE, Harris LS, Friedman MA, Dewey WL, Carchman RA.

Abstract
Oral administration of delta-9-THC (25-100 mg/kg) bound to bovine serum albumin was investigated for potential antitumor action on Lewis lung carcinoma. BDG1 male mice were inoculated with 106 tumor cells into right hind leg and treated daily for 10 days beginning 24 hrs. after tumor implantation. On day 12 of this experiment , delta-9-THC

retarded primarytumor growth 48%, 72% and 75% at 25, 50 and 100 mg/kg, respectively. Mice receiving 100 mg/kg survived 36% longer than control as compared to 45% for the cyclophosphamide positive control. Mice treated for 20 days showed slightly less inhibition of primary tumor growth with no increase in lifespan. In this study, cannabinol, at the same doses at delta-9-THC. administered for 20 days showed slightly less activity on tumor growth and did not prolong survival time. In preliminary mechanismistic studies, delta-9-THC administered acutely, inhibited 3H thymidine uptake into tumor DNA but not in brain, testes, spleen or bone marrow. Twenty-four hours after a single oral gavage of 400 mg/kg delta-9-THC, DNA synthesis was reduced 75%. DNA synthesis was not significantly altered in primary tumor or tissues of mice similarly treated for 20 days.

Link: https://archives.drugabuse.gov/pdf/monographs/01.pdf

From: **Findings of Drug Abuse Research**, a publication of the National Institute of Drug Abuse, 1976

1976

Retardation of Tumor Growth
Marihuana Research Findings: 1976
Editor, Robert C. Petersen, Ph.D.
NIDA RESEARCH MONOGRAPH

"Harris et al. (1976) have reported that mice innoculated with Lewis lung adenocarcinoma showed tumor size reductions ranging from 25-82 percent depending on the dose and duration of treatment with oral - 8-THC, -9-THC and cannabinol. No reductions were found with cannabidiol. The effective cannabinoids increased survival time from one-quarter to one-third compared to a 50 percent increase with cyclophosphamide. Friend leukemia virus growth was inhibited by -9-THC, but L1210 murine leukemia was not. In vitro experiments confirmed the inhibition of neoplastic growth in mice, leading the authors to conclude that certain cannabinoids possess antineoplastic properties by virtue of their interference with RNA and DNA synthesis. In a later study (Harris, 1976), other tumor systems and other cannabinoids were tested. He found that cannabidiol seems to have a growth-enhancing, rather than reducing, effect on the Lewis lung tumor. White et al. (1976), working with Lewis lung cell cultures exposed to -9-THC concluded that at non-toxic doses, the drug inhibits replication after thymidine uptake. This cytotoxicity may be related to -9-THC's extreme lipophilia, and, therefore, the results are related to effects on membrane function."

Link: https://archives.drugabuse.gov/pdf/monographs/14.pdf

In vivo effects of cannabinoids on macromolecular biosynthesis in Lewis lung carcinomas.
Cancer Biochemistry Biophysics
Friedman MA.

Abstract

Cannabinoids represent a novel class of drugs active in increasing the life span mice carrying Lewis lung tumors and decreasing primary tumor size. In the present studies, the effects of delta9-THC, delta8-THC, and cannabidiol on tumor macromolecular biosynthesis were studied. These drugs inhibit thymidine-3H incorporation into DNA acutely, but did not inhibit leucine uptake into tumor protein. At 24 h after treatment, cannabinoids did not inhibit thymidine-3H incorporation into DNA, leucine-3H uptake into protein or cytidine-3H into RNA.

PubMed Link: http://www.ncbi.nlm.nih.gov/pubmed/616322

Between 1977, and 1990, no pre clinical studies can be found that demonstrate substances in marijuana can kill cancer cells. There was no follow up by our government to the studies quoted above, yet hundreds of thousands of dollars were invested in *other* attempts to find a cancer cure. *However, after the discovery of the endocannabinoid system in 1990, researchers in the lab began to rediscover this again.*

Inhibition by delta-9-tetrahydrocannabinol of tumor necrosis factor alpha production by mouse and human macrophages.
International Journal of Immunopharmacology

Zheng ZM, Specter S, Friedman H.
Department of Medical Microbiology and Immunology, University of South Florida College of Medicine, Tampa

Abstract

Suppression by delta-9-tetrahydrocannabinol (THC) of tumor necrosis factor (TNF) production by macrophages has not been reported previously. The present study evaluated the effect in vitro of THC on soluble TNF-alpha production by cultured murine peritoneal macrophages. THC at 5 or 10 micrograms/ml added to medium [RPMI 1640 containing 10 ng LPS/ml, mouse IFN-gamma (100 u/ml), and 0.5% bovine serum albumin (BSA)] used to induce TNF significantly decreased TNF-alpha production by BALB/c mouse macrophages. Macrophages pretreated with THC at 0.1, 0.5, or 1.0 micrograms/ml in protein-free medium for 3 h at 37 degrees C, prior to TNF induction, also showed a decreased ability to produce TNF-alpha in a dose-dependent manner. Increasing the protein concentration from 0.5 to 5% BSA in the medium which was used to induce TNF prevented the inhibitory activity of THC. Human peripheral blood adherent cells treated with THC-containing medium produced less TNF-alpha than controls that were not exposed to THC. Thus, our data provide evidence that THC can inhibit TNF production by mouse and human macrophages. The drug's activity is concentration dependent and is related to the amount of serum protein in the medium used to induce this cytokine.

PubMed Link: http://www.ncbi.nlm.nih.gov/pubmed/1334476

1993

Delta-9-Tetrahydrocannabinol inhibits cell contact-dependent cytotoxicity of Bacillus Calmétte-Guérin-activated macrophages.

International Journal of Immunopharmacology

Burnette-Curley D, Marciano-Cabral F, Fischer-Stenger K, Cabral GA.
Medical College of Virginia/Virginia Commonwealth University, Department of Microbiology and Immunology, Richmond.

Abstract

The effect of delta-9-tetrahydrocannabinol (delta-9-THC), the major psychoactive component of marijuana, on the capacity of Bacillus Calmétte-Guérin (BCG)-activated macrophages to lyse L929 tumor cells, Naegleria fowleri amoebae, and herpes simplex virus-infected cells was examined. Delta-9-THC inhibited tumoricidal and amoebicidal activity in a dose-related manner. Antiviral activity was decreased when mice received 25 and 50 mg/kg delta-9-THC. The cannabinoid did not directly suppress the activation of macrophages as determined by levels of 5'-nucleotidase activity and did not inhibit splenic T-lymphocytes of BCG-recipient mice from producing interferon gamma. Nomarski optics microscopy, scanning electron microscopy, and radiolabeling binding studies demonstrated that macrophages from delta-9-THC-treated mice retained their capacity to attach to their targets. These results suggest that delta-9-THC suppresses cell contact-dependent amoebicidal, tumoricidal, and antiviral activities of activated macrophages at a stage following effector cell-target cell conjugation.

PubMed Link: http://www.ncbi.nlm.nih.gov/pubmed/8389327

Delta 9-tetrahydrocannabinol inhibition of tumor necrosis factor-alpha: suppression of post-translational events.

Journal of Pharmacology and Experimental Theraputics

Fischer-Stenger K, Dove Pettit DA, Cabral GA.
Department of Microbiology and Immunology, Medical College of Virginia/Virginia Commonwealth University, Richmond.

Abstract
Delta 9-tetrahydrocannabinol (delta 9-THC), the major psychoactive component of marijuana, has been shown to suppress macrophage soluble cytolytic activity. The purpose of this study was to determine whether delta 9-THC inhibited this function by affecting tumor necrosis factor-alpha (TNF-alpha). The RAW264.7 macrophage cell line was used as an in vitro bacterial lipopolysaccharide-inducible system for production of TNF-alpha. Macrophage-conditioned medium of RAW264.7 macrophages treated with delta 9-THC was shown to be deficient in tumoricidal activity. Immunoprecipitation experiments demonstrated that the macrophage-conditioned medium of cultures treated with drug contained lower levels of TNF-alpha. Northern analysis indicated that delta 9-THC had no effect on the levels of TNF-alpha messenger RNA. However, radiolabel pulsing and pulse-chase experiments revealed that the intracellular conversion of the 26-kD presecreted form of TNF-alpha to the 17-kD secreted form was inhibited by the drug. These results indicate that delta 9-THC suppresses soluble macrophage tumoricidal activity, at least in part, by decreasing the intracellular conversion of presecretory TNF-alpha to its 17-kD secretory form.

PubMed Link: http://www.ncbi.nlm.nih.gov/pubmed/8263818

1995

Differential inhibition of RAW264.7 macrophage tumoricidal activity by delta 9tetrahydrocannabinol.

Proceedings of the Society for Experimental Biology and Medicine

Burnette-Curley D, Cabral GA.
Department of Microbiology and Immunology, Virginia Commonwealth University/Medical College of Virginia, Richmond, USA.

Abstract
delta 9tetrahydrocannabinol (THC), the major psychoactive component of marijuana, has been shown to inhibit macrophage cell contact-dependent cytolysis of tumor cells. The purpose of this study was to determine whether THC inhibited macrophage cytolytic function by targeting selectively tumor necrosis factor (TNF)-dependent pathways versus L-arginine-dependent reactive nitrogen intermediates. An in vitro system employing RAW264.7 macrophage-like cells as effectors and TNF-sensitive mouse L929 fibroblasts or nitric oxide (NO.)-sensitive P815 mastocytoma cells as targets, was employed to assess the effect of THC on cytolysis. Macrophages were pretreated with THC or vehicle for 48 hr, subjected to multistep activation with 10 U/ml recombinant mouse gamma-interferon

(IFN-gamma) plus 100 ng/ml LPS or to direct activation with 1 microgram/ml LPS, and co-cultured with tumor cells in the presence or absence of THC. THC inhibited TNF-dependent killing by macrophages subjected to either multistep or direct activation. Decreased amounts of TNF-alpha were detected in medium of macrophage cultures treated with THC. In contrast, THC inhibited NO.-dependent cell contact killing only for macrophages subjected to direct activation. Decreased levels of NO2-, a stable degradation product of the short-lived and highly toxic effector molecule NO., were produced by these macrophages. In addition, the effect of the enantiomeric pairs (-)CP55,940/(+)CP56,667 or (-)HU-210/(+)HU-211 on macrophage cell contact-dependent killing was assessed. Inhibition of macrophage tumoricidal activity against TNF-sensitive L929 cells was effected by both isomers of THC analogs. In contrast, both of the enantiomeric pairs had an effect on killing of NO.-sensitive P815 mastocytoma cells only for macrophages subjected to direct activation. These data suggest that cannabinoids inhibit macrophage cell contact-dependent killing of tumor cells by a noncannabinoid receptor-mediated mechanism. However, specific cytolytic pathways are inhibited differentially by cannabinoids depending on the activation stimuli to which macrophages are exposed.

PubMed Link: http://www.ncbi.nlm.nih.gov/pubmed/7675800

1996

Delta-9-tetrahydrocannabinol suppresses tumor necrosis factor alpha maturation and secretion but not its transcription in mouse macrophages.

International Journal of Immunopharmacology

Zheng ZM, Specter SC.
Department of Medical Microbiology and Immunology, University of South Florida, College of Medicine, Tampa, USA.

Abstract
Various in vitro studies have shown that delta-9-tetrahydrocannabinol (THC), the major psychoactive component of marijuana, has a variety of inhibitory effects on immune functions including effects on macrophages. The present studies have examined the mechanism of THC's effects on tumor necrosis factor alpha (TNF-alpha), a major macrophage-produced cytokine and an important mediator involved in cytokine networks and in host defense mechanisms. Exposure of macrophages to medium containing THC has resulted in low levels of soluble TNF-alpha protein and reduced TNF-alpha bioactivity in the culture supernatant. However, THC did not inhibit the levels of LPS-induced TNF-alpha mRNA and intracellular TNF-alpha precursor protein, had only a weak effect on expression of membrane-bound TNF-alpha, but suppressed TNF-alpha maturation/secretion by macrophages. The higher the THC concentration in the medium during TNF-alpha induction, the greater the amount of intracellular TNF-alpha precursors that accumulated in the activated macrophages and the less mature TNF-alpha was released from the cells. Data suggest that TNF-alpha production by macrophages was altered greatly by exposure to THC at the levels of TNF-alpha precursor maturation and secretion.

PubMed Link: http://www.ncbi.nlm.nih.gov/pubmed/8732433

2000

Anti-tumoral action of cannabinoids: involvement of sustained ceramide accumulation and extracellular signal-regulated kinase activation.

Nature Medicine

Galve-Roperh I, Sánchez C, Cortés ML, Gómez del Pulgar T, Izquierdo M, Guzmán M.
Department of Biochemistry and Molecular Biology I, School of Biology, Complutense University, Madrid, Spain.

Abstract
Delta9-Tetrahydrocannabinol, the main active component of marijuana, induces apoptosis of transformed neural cells in culture. Here, we show that intratumoral administration of Delta9-tetrahydrocannabinol and the synthetic cannabinoid agonist WIN-55,212-2 induced a considerable regression of malignant gliomas in Wistar rats and in mice deficient in recombination activating gene 2. Cannabinoid treatment did not produce any substantial neurotoxic effect in the conditions used. Experiments with two subclones of C6 glioma cells in culture showed that cannabinoids signal apoptosis by a pathway involving cannabinoid receptors, sustained ceramide accumulation and Raf1/extracellular signal-regulated kinase activation. These results may provide the basis for a new therapeutic approach for the treatment of malignant gliomas.

PubMed Link: http://www.ncbi.nlm.nih.gov/pubmed/10700234

also: Pot of gold for glioma therapy.
http://www.nature.com/nm/journal/v6/n3/full/nm0300_255.html

2001

Inhibition of glioma growth in vivo by selective activation of the CB(2) cannabinoid receptor.

Cancer Research

Sánchez C, de Ceballos ML, Gomez del Pulgar T, Rueda D, Corbacho C, Velasco G, Galve-Roperh I, Huffman JW, Ramón y Cajal S, Guzmán M.
Department of Biochemistry and Molecular Biology I, School of Biology, Complutense University, Madrid, Spain.

Abstract
The development of new therapeutic strategies is essential for the management of gliomas, one of the most malignant forms of cancer. We have shown previously that the growth of the rat glioma C6 cell line is inhibited by psychoactive cannabinoids (I. Galve-Roperh et al., Nat. Med., 6: 313-319, 2000). These compounds act on the brain and some other organs through the widely expressed CB(1) receptor. By contrast, the other cannabinoid receptor

subtype, the CB(2) receptor, shows a much more restricted distribution and is absent from normal brain. Here we show that local administration of the selective CB(2) agonist JWH-133 at 50 microg/day to Rag-2(-/-) mice induced a considerable regression of malignant tumors generated by inoculation of C6 glioma cells. The selective involvement of the CB(2) receptor in this action was evidenced by: (a) the prevention by the CB(2) antagonist SR144528 but not the CB(1) antagonist SR141716; (b) the down-regulation of the CB(2) receptor but not the CB(1) receptor in the tumors; and (c) the absence of typical CB(1)-mediated psychotropic side effects. Cannabinoid receptor expression was subsequently examined in biopsies from human astrocytomas. A full 70% (26 of 37) of the human astrocytomas analyzed expressed significant levels of cannabinoid receptors. Of interest, the extent of CB(2) receptor expression was directly related with tumor malignancy. In addition, the growth of grade IV human astrocytoma cells in Rag-2(-/-) mice was completely blocked by JWH-133 administration at 50 microg/day. Experiments carried out with C6 glioma cells in culture evidenced the internalization of the CB(2) but not the CB(1) receptor upon JWH-133 challenge and showed that selective activation of the CB(2) receptor signaled apoptosis via enhanced ceramide synthesis de novo. These results support a therapeutic approach for the treatment of malignant gliomas devoid of psychotropic side effects.

PubMed Link: http://www.ncbi.nlm.nih.gov/pubmed/11479216

FROM FULL TEXT:

"Marijuana and its derivatives have been used in medicine for many centuries, and nowadays, there is a renaissance in the study of the therapeutic effects of cannabinoids, which constitutes a widely debated issue with ample scientific and social relevance. Ongoing research is determining whether cannabinoid ligands may be effective agents in the treatment of pain (12, 13), glaucoma (14), neuro-degenerative disorders such as Parkinson's disease (15) and multiple sclerosis (16), and the wasting and emesis associated with AIDS and cancer chemotherapy (14). In addition, cannabinoids might be potential antitumoral agents because of their ability to inhibit the growth of various types of cancer cells in culture (17–19). Moreover, in laboratory animals, cannabinoids induce the regression of gliomas, one of the most malignant forms of cancer whose current treatment in patients is usually ineffective or just palliative (20). This growth-inhibiting effect was exerted by two psychoactive cannabinoids, namely THC,4 the main active component of marijuana, and WIN-55,212-2, a nonselective synthetic cannabinoid agonist, pointing to the involvement of cannabinoid receptors (20)."

Complete Study:
http://cancerres.aacrjournals.org/content/61/15/5784.full.pdf

2003

Inhibition of skin tumor growth and angiogenesis in vivo by activation of cannabinoid receptors.

Journal of Clinical Investigation

Casanova ML, Blázquez C, Martínez-Palacio J, Villanueva C, Fernández-Aceñero MJ, Huffman JW, Jorcano JL, Guzmán M.
Project on Cellular and Molecular Biology and Gene Therapy, Centro de Investigaciones Energéticas, Medioambientales y Tecnológicas, Madrid, Spain.

Abstract

Nonmelanoma skin cancer is one of the most common malignancies in humans. Different therapeutic strategies for the treatment of these tumors are currently being investigated. Given the growth-inhibiting effects of cannabinoids on gliomas and the wide tissue distribution of the two subtypes of cannabinoid receptors (CB(1) and CB(2)), we studied the potential utility of these compounds in anti-skin tumor therapy. Here we show that the CB(1) and the CB(2) receptor are expressed in normal skin and skin tumors of mice and humans. In cell culture experiments pharmacological activation of cannabinoid receptors induced the apoptotic death of tumorigenic epidermal cells, whereas the viability of nontransformed epidermal cells remained unaffected. Local administration of the mixed CB(1)/CB(2) agonist WIN-55,212-2 or the selective CB(2) agonist JWH-133 induced a considerable growth inhibition of malignant tumors generated by inoculation of epidermal tumor cells into nude mice. Cannabinoid-treated tumors showed an increased number of apoptotic cells. This was accompanied by impairment of tumor vascularization, as determined by altered blood vessel morphology and decreased expression of proangiogenic factors (VEGF, placental growth factor, and angiopoietin 2). Abrogation of EGF-R function was also observed in cannabinoid-treated tumors. These results support a new therapeutic approach for the treatment of skin tumors.

PubMed Link: https://www.ncbi.nlm.nih.gov/pubmed/12511587

New Toke on Treating Skin Cancer
Lab Animal
March 2003

"The active components in marijuana inhibit the growth of nonmelanoma skin tumors in mice, with no inhalation necessary, suggesting that cannabinoids may be a potential therapy for one of the most common malignancies in humans... Risk factors for nonmelanoma skin cancers include fair skin and excessive sun exposure."

http://www.labanimal.com/laban/journal/v32/n3/pdf/laban0303-12b.pdf

Complete Study:
On Pub Med:
https://www.ncbi.nlm.nih.gov/pubmed/12630416

Inhibition of tumor angiogenesis by cannabinoids

Federation of Experimental Biology

Blázquez C, Casanova ML, Planas A, Gómez Del Pulgar T, Villanueva C, Fernández-Aceñero MJ, Aragonés J, Huffman JW, Jorcano JL, Guzmán M.

Department of Biochemistry and Molecular Biology I, School of Biology, Complutense University, Madrid, Spain.

Abstract

Cannabinoids, the active components of marijuana and their derivatives, induce tumor regression in rodents (8). However, the mechanism of cannabinoid antitumoral action in vivo is as yet unknown. Here we show that local administration of a nonpsychoactive cannabinoid to mice inhibits angiogenesis of malignant gliomas as determined by immunohistochemical analyses and vascular permeability assays. In vitro and in vivo experiments show that at least two mechanisms may be involved in this cannabinoid action: the direct inhibition of vascular endothelial cell migration and survival as well as the decrease of the expression of proangiogenic factors (vascular endothelial growth factor and angiopoietin-2) and matrix metalloproteinase-2 in the tumors. Inhibition of tumor angiogenesis may allow new strategies for the design of cannabinoid-based antitumoral therapies.

PubMed Link: https://www.ncbi.nlm.nih.gov/pubmed/12514108

Cannabinoids: potential anticancer agents.

Nature Reviews. Cancer.

Guzmán M

Department of Biochemistry and Molecular Biology I, School of Biology, Complutense University, Madrid, Spain.

Abstract

Cannabinoids - the active components of Cannabis sativa and their derivatives - exert palliative effects in cancer patients by preventing nausea, vomiting and pain and by stimulating appetite. In addition, these compounds have been shown to inhibit the growth of tumour cells in culture and animal models by modulating key cell-signalling pathways. Cannabinoids are usually well tolerated, and do not produce the generalized toxic effects of conventional chemotherapies. So, could cannabinoids be used to develop new anticancer therapies?

PubMed Link: https://www.ncbi.nlm.nih.gov/pubmed/14570037

Cannabinoid receptor systems: therapeutic targets for tumour intervention.

Expert Opinion on Theraputic Targets

Jones S, Howl J.
Molecular Pharmacology Group, Biomedical Sciences Division, School of Applied Sciences, University of Wolverhampton, UK.

The past decade has witnessed a rapid expansion of our understanding of the biological roles of cannabinoids and their cognate receptors. It is now certain that Delta9-tetrahydrocannabinol, the principle psychoactive component of the Cannabis sativa plant, binds and activates membrane receptors of the 7-transmembrane domain, G-protein-coupled super-family. Several putative endocannabinoids have since been identified, including anandamide, 2-arachidonyl glycerol and noladin ether. Synthesis of numerous cannabinomimetics has also greatly expanded the repertoire of cannabinoid receptor ligands with the pharmacodynamic properties of agonists, antagonists and inverse agonists. Collectively, these ligands have proven to be powerful tools both for the molecular characterisation of cannabinoid receptors and the delineation of their intrinsic signalling pathways. Much of our understanding of the signalling mechanisms activated by cannabinoids is derived from studies of receptors expressed by tumour cells; hence, this review provides a succinct summary of the molecular pharmacology of cannabinoid receptors and their roles in tumour cell biology. Moreover, there is now a genuine expectation that the manipulation of cannabinoid receptor systems may have therapeutic potential for a diverse range of human diseases. Thus, this review also summarises the demonstrated antitumour actions of cannabinoids and indicates possible avenues for the future development of cannabinoids as antitumour agents.

PubMed Link: http://www.ncbi.nlm.nih.gov/pubmed/14640910

2004

Cannabinoids inhibit the vascular endothelial growth factor pathway in gliomas.

Cancer Research

Blázquez C, González-Feria L, Alvarez L, Haro A, Casanova ML, Guzmán M.
Department of Biochemistry and Molecular Biology I, School of Biology, Complutense University, Madrid, Spain.

Abstract
Cannabinoids inhibit tumor angiogenesis in mice, but the mechanism of their antiangiogenic action is still unknown. Because the vascular endothelial growth factor (VEGF) pathway plays a critical role in tumor angiogenesis, here we studied whether cannabinoids affect it. As a first approach, cDNA array analysis showed that cannabinoid administration to mice bearing s.c. gliomas lowered the expression of various VEGF pathway-related genes. The use of other methods (ELISA, Western blotting, and confocal microscopy)

provided additional evidence that cannabinoids depressed the VEGF pathway by decreasing the production of VEGF and the activation of VEGF receptor (VEGFR)-2, the most prominent VEGF receptor, in cultured glioma cells and in mouse gliomas. Cannabinoid-induced inhibition of VEGF production and VEGFR-2 activation was abrogated both in vitro and in vivo by pharmacological blockade of ceramide biosynthesis. These changes in the VEGF pathway were paralleled by changes in tumor size. Moreover, intratumoral administration of the cannabinoid Delta9-tetrahydrocannabinol to two patients with glioblastoma multiforme (grade IV astrocytoma) decreased VEGF levels and VEGFR-2 activation in the tumors. Because blockade of the VEGF pathway constitutes one of the most promising antitumoral approaches currently available, the present findings provide a novel pharmacological target for cannabinoid-based therapies.

PubMed Link: https://www.ncbi.nlm.nih.gov/pubmed/15313899

Antitumor effects of cannabidiol, a nonpsychoactive cannabinoid, on human glioma cell lines.

Journal of Pharmacology and Experimental Therapeutics

Massi P, Vaccani A, Ceruti S, Colombo A,
Abbracchio MP, Parolaro D.
Department of Pharmacology, University of Milan, Milan, Italy.

Abstract

Recently, cannabinoids (CBs) have been shown to possess antitumor properties. Because the psychoactivity of cannabinoid compounds limits their medicinal usage, we undertook the present study to evaluate the in vitro antiproliferative ability of cannabidiol (CBD), a nonpsychoactive cannabinoid compound, on U87 and U373 human glioma cell lines. The addition of CBD to the culture medium led to a dramatic drop of mitochondrial oxidative metabolism [3-(4,5-dimethyl-2-thiazolyl)-2,5-diphenyl-2H tetrazolium bromide test] and viability in glioma cells, in a concentration-dependent manner that was already evident 24 h after CBD exposure, with an apparent IC(50) of 25 microM. The antiproliferative effect of CBD was partially prevented by the CB2 receptor antagonist N-[(1S)-endo-1,3,3-trimethylbicyclo[2,2,1]heptan-2-yl]-5-(4-chloro-3-methylphenyl)-1-(4-methylbenzyl)-pyrazole-3-carboxamide (SR144528; SR2) and alpha-tocopherol. By contrast, the CB1 cannabinoid receptor antagonist N-(piperidin-1-yl)-5-(4-chlorophenyl)-1-(2,4-dichlorophenyl)-4-methyl-1H-pyrazole-3-carboximide hydrochloride (SR141716; SR1), capsazepine (vanilloid receptor antagonist), the inhibitors of ceramide generation, or pertussis toxin did not counteract CBD effects. We also show, for the first time, that the antiproliferative effect of CBD was correlated to induction of apoptosis, as determined by cytofluorimetric analysis and single-strand DNA staining, which was not reverted by cannabinoid antagonists. Finally, CBD, administered s.c. to nude mice at the dose of 0.5 mg/mouse, significantly inhibited the growth of subcutaneously implanted U87 human glioma cells. In conclusion, the nonpsychoactive CBD was able to produce a significant antitumor activity both in vitro and in vivo, thus suggesting a possible application of CBD as an antineoplastic agent.

PubMed Link: https://www.ncbi.nlm.nih.gov/pubmed/14617682

FROM FULL TEXT:

"Marijuana and its derivatives have been used in medicine for many centuries, and currently there is a renewed interest in the study of the therapeutic effects of cannabinoids. Cannabinoids produce their effects by binding to specific plasma membrane G protein-coupled receptors. To date, two cannabinoid receptors have been characterized: the CB1 receptor, expressed primarily in the brain and in some peripheral tissues, and CB2 receptors, expressed by cells of the immune system (Howlett et al., 2002; Pertwee and Ross, 2002). Ongoing research is determining whether cannabinoid ligands may be effective agents in the treatment of pain, glaucoma, the wasting and emesis associated with cancer chemotherapy and AIDS, and neurodegenerative disorders such as multiple sclerosis (Gouto-poulos and Makriyannis, 2002). Among the potential therapeutic activities, one of the most exciting and promising areas of current cannabinoid research is the demonstrated ability of these compounds to affect a number of pathways involved in the cell survival/death decision (Bifulco and Di Marzo, 2002; Guzman et al., 2002).

Both natural and synthetic as well as endogenous cannabinoids have been found to affect the rate of cell proliferation in cell lines derived from the central nervous system. Very intriguing was the demonstration that THC and WIN-55,212-2 have been demonstrated to suppress the growth of rat glioma C6 cells inoculated intracerebrally in the rat or subcutaneously in immune-deficient mice, through a cannabinoid receptor-dependent mechanism (Sanchez et al., 1998; Galve-Roperh et al., 2000; Guzman et al., 2002)."

Complete Study:
http://jpet.aspetjournals.org/content/308/3/838.long

Hypothesis: cannabinoid therapy for the treatment of gliomas?

Neuropharmacology

Velasco G, Galve-Roperh I, Sánchez C, Blázquez C, Guzmán M.
Department of Biochemistry and Molecular Biology I, School of Biology, Complutense University, Madrid, Spain.

Abstract

Gliomas, in particular glioblastoma multiforme or grade IV astrocytoma, are the most frequent class of malignant primary brain tumours and one of the most aggressive forms of cancer. Current therapeutic strategies for the treatment of glioblastoma multiforme are usually ineffective or just palliative. During the last few years, several studies have shown that cannabinoids-the active components of the plant Cannabis sativa and their derivatives--slow the growth of different types of tumours, including gliomas, in laboratory animals. Cannabinoids induce apoptosis of glioma cells in culture via sustained ceramide accumulation, extracellular signal-regulated kinase activation and Akt inhibition. In addition, cannabinoid treatment inhibits angiogenesis of gliomas in vivo. Remarkably, cannabinoids kill glioma cells selectively and can protect non-transformed glial cells from death. These and other findings reviewed here might set the basis for a potential use of cannabinoids in the management of gliomas.

PubMed Link: https://www.ncbi.nlm.nih.gov/pubmed/15275820

FROM FULL TEXT:

"The hemp plant Cannabis sativa produces approximately 60 unique compounds known as cannabinoids, of which D9-tetrahydrocannabinol (THC) is the most studied owing to its high potency and abundance in cannabis (Gaoni and Mechoulam, 1964) ... THC exerts a wide variety of biological effects by mimicking endogenous substances—the endocannabinoids anandamide and 2-arachidonoylglycerol (Fig. 1)—that bind to and activate specific cannabinoid receptors... Apart from these palliative actions, a number of plant-derived (for example, THC and cannabidiol), synthetic (for example, WIN-55,212-2 and HU-210) and endogenous cannabinoids (for example, anandamide and 2-arachidonoylglycerol) have been shown to exert antiproliferative actions on a wide spectrum of tumour cells in culture."

Complete Study:
https://www.researchgate.net/publication/8433601_Hypothesis_Cannabin oid_therapy_for_the_treatment_of_gliomas

2005

Cannabidiol inhibits human glioma cell migration through a cannabinoid receptor-independent mechanism.

British Journal of Pharmacology
Vaccani A, Massi P, Colombo A, Rubino T, Parolaro D.
Department of Structural and Functional Biology, Pharmacology Section, Center of Neurosciences, University of Insubria, Italy.

Abstract
We evaluated the ability of cannabidiol (CBD) to impair the migration of tumor cells stimulated by conditioned medium. CBD caused concentration-dependent inhibition of the migration of U87 glioma cells, quantified in a Boyden chamber. Since these cells express both cannabinoid CB1 and CB2 receptors in the membrane, we also evaluated their engagement in the antimigratory effect of CBD. The inhibition of cell was not antagonized either by the selective cannabinoid receptor antagonists SR141716 (CB1) and SR144528 (CB2) or by pretreatment with pertussis toxin, indicating no involvement of classical cannabinoid receptors and/or receptors coupled to Gi/o proteins. These results reinforce the evidence of antitumoral properties of CBD, demonstrating its ability to limit tumor invasion, although the mechanism of its pharmacological effects remains to be clarified.

PubMed Link: https://www.ncbi.nlm.nih.gov/pubmed/15700028

FROM FULL TEXT:

"Malignant gliomas are highly infiltrating, proliferative tumors. Glioma cells follow a characteristic pattern of growth, invading the adjacent normal brain structures and surrounding large blood vessels. Inhibiting migration is therefore a vital step towards improving the prognosis of patients with malignant gliomas. In a previous study, we demonstrated that CBD, a nonpsychotropic derivative of marijuana, impaired the viability of human glioma cell lines U87 and U373 in vitro and in vivo, suggesting its potential medical use."

Complete Study:

https://www.ncbi.nlm.nih.gov/pmc/articles/PMC1576089/

Cannabinoids selectively inhibit proliferation and induce death of cultured human glioblastoma multiforme cells.

Journal of Neuro-oncology.
McAllister SD, Chan C, Taft RJ,
Luu T, Abood ME, Moore DH, Aldape K, Yount G.
California Pacific Medical Center Research Institute,

Abstract

Normal tissue toxicity limits the efficacy of current treatment modalities for glioblastoma multiforme (GBM). We evaluated the influence of cannabinoids on cell proliferation, death, and morphology of human GBM cell lines and in primary human glial cultures, the normal cells from which GBM tumors arise. The influence of a plant derived cannabinoid agonist, Delta(9)-tetrahydrocannabinol Delta(9)-THC), and a potent synthetic cannabinoid agonist, WIN 55,212-2, were compared using time lapse microscopy. We discovered that Delta(9)-THC decreases cell proliferation and increases cell death of human GBM cells more rapidly than WIN 55,212-2. Delta(9)-THC was also more potent at inhibiting the proliferation of GBM cells compared to WIN 55,212-2. The effects of Delta(9)-THC and WIN 55,212-2 on the GBM cells were partially the result of cannabinoid receptor activation. The same concentration of Delta(9)-THC that significantly inhibits proliferation and increases death of human GBM cells has no significant impact on human primary glial cultures. Evidence of selective efficacy with WIN 55,212-2 was also observed but the selectivity was less profound, and the synthetic agonist produced a greater disruption of normal cell morphology compared to Delta(9)-THC.

PubMed Link: https://www.ncbi.nlm.nih.gov/pubmed/16078104

FROM FULL TEXT:

"Cannabinoids have been shown to control cell growth and death in multiple types of cancer [1]. The endocannabinoid system was discovered through research focusing on the primary active component of Cannabis sativa, D9-THC, and other synthetic cannabinoids [2]. To date, two G-protein coupled receptors, CB1 and CB2, have been demonstrated to mediate a majority of the pharmacological effects of the compounds...cannabinoids have been shown to produce direct antiproliferative and apoptotic effects in cell lines derived from many types of cancers [6]. This direct antitumor activity has been primarily attributed to the activation of both CB1 and CB2 receptors but there is also data suggesting that cannabinoids can directly inhibit the growth of cancer through other mechanisms [7,8]. The possibility that cannabinoids might also inhibit tumor growth indirectly is supported by studies demonstrating that cannabinoid compounds can decrease angiogenesis through modulation of proangiogenic factors [9,10]. Of potential clinical relevance is the selective efficacy apparent with cannabinoids. Compounds activating the endocannabinoid system can induce apoptosis in rat C6 glioma cells in vitro as well as inhibit growth and eradicate tumors in vivo [11]. Importantly, cannabinoid-induced cell death was observed in C6 glioma cells but this phenomenon was not seen in rodent primary astrocytes and neuronal cultures [12]. This finding was further supported by in vivo data showing cannabinoids could inhibit, and in some cases eradicate, C6 glioma tumors but there was no discernable tissue damage in surrounding healthy tissue [11]."

Complete Study Link:

http://theroc.us/images/Cannabinoids%20selectively%20inhibit%20prolife
ration%20and%20induce%20death%20of%20cultured%20human%20glio
blastoma%20multiforme%20cells.pdf

Targeting cannabinoid receptors to treat leukemia: role of cross-talk between extrinsic and intrinsic pathways in Delta9-tetrahydrocannabinol (THC)-induced apoptosis of Jurkat cells.

Leukemia Research.
Lombard C, Nagarkatti M, Nagarkatti PS.
Department of Microbiology and Immunology, Medical College of Virginia Campus, Virginia Commonwealth University, Richmond, VA, USA.

Abstract

Targeting cannabinoid receptors has recently been shown to trigger apoptosis and offers a novel treatment modality against malignancies of the immune system. However, the precise mechanism of apoptosis in such cancers has not been previously addressed. In this study, we used human Jurkat leukemia cell lines with defects in intrinsic and extrinsic signaling pathways to elucidate the mechanism of apoptosis induced by Delta9-tetrahydrocannabinol (THC). We observed that Jurkat cells deficient in FADD or caspase-8 were partially resistant to apoptosis, while dominant-negative caspase-9 mutant cells were completely resistant to apoptosis. Use of caspase inhibitors confirmed these results. Furthermore, overexpression of Bcl-2 rendered the cells resistant to THC at early time points but not upon prolonged exposure. THC treatment led to loss of Deltapsi(m), in both wild-type and FADD-deficient Jurkat cells thereby suggesting that THC-induced intrinsic pathway was independent of FADD. THC treatment of wild-type Jurkat cells caused cytochrome c release, and cleavage of caspase-8, -9, -2, -10, and Bid. Caspase-2 inhibitor blocked THC-induced caspase-3 in wild-type Jurkat cells but not loss of Deltapsi(m). Together, these data suggest that the intrinsic pathway plays a more critical role in THC-induced apoptosis while the extrinsic pathway may facilitate apoptosis via cross-talk with the intrinsic pathway.

PubMed Link: https://www.ncbi.nlm.nih.gov/pubmed/15978942

Cannabinoids and cancer: potential for colorectal cancer therapy.

Biochemical Society Transactions.

Patsos HA, Hicks DJ, Greenhough A, Williams AC, Paraskeva C.
Cancer Research UK Colorectal Tumour Biology Group, Department of Cellular and Molecular Medicine, School of Medical Sciences, University of Bristol, Bristol, UK.

Abstract
Despite extensive research into the biology of CRC (colorectal cancer), and recent advances in surgical techniques and chemotherapy, CRC continues to be a major cause of death throughout the world. Therefore it is important to develop novel chemopreventive/chemotherapeutic agents for CRC. Cannabinoids are a class of compounds that are currently used in the treatment of chemotherapy-induced nausea and vomiting, and in the stimulation of appetite. However, there is accumulating evidence that they could also be useful for the inhibition of tumour cell growth by modulating key survival signalling pathways. The chemotherapeutic potential for plant-derived and endogenous cannabinoids in CRC therapy is reviewed.

PubMed Link: https://www.ncbi.nlm.nih.gov/pubmed/16042581

Cannabis-induced cytotoxicity in leukemic cell lines: the role of the cannabinoid receptors and the MAPK pathway.

Blood.

Powles T, te Poele R, Shamash J, Chaplin T, Propper D, Joel S, Oliver T, Liu WM.
New Drug Study Group, St. Bartholomew's Hospital, London, United Kingdom.

Abstract
Delta9-Tetrahydrocannabinol (THC) is the active metabolite of cannabis. THC causes cell death in vitro through the activation of complex signal transduction pathways. However, the role that the cannabinoid 1 and 2 receptors (CB1-R and CB2-R) play in this process is less clear. We therefore investigated the role of the CB-Rs in mediating apoptosis in 3 leukemic cell lines and performed microarray and immunoblot analyses to establish further the mechanism of cell death. We developed a novel flow cytometric technique of measuring the expression of functional receptors and used combinations of selective CB1-R and

CB2-R antagonists and agonists to determine their individual roles in this process. We have shown that THC is a potent inducer of apoptosis, even at 1 x IC(50) (inhibitory concentration 50%) concentrations and as early as 6 hours after exposure to the drug. These effects were seen in leukemic cell lines (CEM, HEL-92, and HL60) as well as in peripheral blood mononuclear cells. Additionally, THC did not appear to act synergistically with cytotoxic agents such as cisplatin. One of the most intriguing findings was that THC-induced cell death was preceded by significant changes in the expression of genes involved in the mitogen-activated protein kinase (MAPK) signal transduction pathways. Both apoptosis and gene expression changes were altered independent of p53 and the CB-Rs.

PubMed Link: https://www.ncbi.nlm.nih.gov/pubmed/15454482

FROM FULL TEXT:
"Δ9-Tetrahydrocannabinol (THC) is the active metabolite of cannabis. Although its analgesic and antiemetic effects in cancer patients has been known for some time, its application has been restricted for social reasons. Interest in this field has intensified with the findings that THC may selectively induce tumor regression both in vitro and in vivo.2-4 Recently, clinical trials using this drug have commenced in Spain. The mechanism underlying its cytotoxic activity has not been elucidated; however, a number of studies have suggested that cannabinoid receptors are involved in this process."

Complete Study Link:
http://www.bloodjournal.org/content/105/3/1214?sso-checked=true

2006

Unheated Cannabis sativa extracts and its major compound THC-acid have potential immuno-modulating properties not mediated by CB1 and CB2 receptor coupled pathways
International Immunopharmacology.

Verhoeckx KC, Korthout HA, van Meeteren-Kreikamp AP, Ehlert KA, Wang M, van der Greef J, Rodenburg RJ, Witkamp RF.
TNO Pharma, Utrechtseweg, PZeist, The Netherlands.

Abstract
There is a great interest in the pharmacological properties of cannabinoid like compounds that are not linked to the adverse effects of Delta(9)-tetrahydrocannabinol (THC), e.g. psychoactive properties. The present paper describes the potential immuno-modulating activity of unheated Cannabis sativa extracts and its main non-psychoactive constituent Delta(9)-tetrahydrocanabinoid acid (THCa). By heating Cannabis extracts, THCa was shown to be converted into THC. Unheated Cannabis extract and THCa were able to inhibit the tumor necrosis factor alpha (TNF-alpha) levels in culture supernatants from

U937 macrophages and peripheral blood macrophages after stimulation with LPS in a dose-dependent manner. This inhibition persisted over a longer period of time, whereas after prolonged exposure time THC and heated Cannabis extract tend to induce the TNF-alpha level. Furthermore we demonstrated that THCa and THC show distinct effects on phosphatidylcholine specific phospholipase C (PC-PLC) activity. Unheated Cannabis extract and THCa inhibit the PC-PLC activity in a dose-dependent manner, while THC induced PC-PLC activity at high concentrations. These results suggest that THCa and THC exert their immuno-modulating effects via different metabolic pathways.

PubMed Link: https://www.ncbi.nlm.nih.gov/pubmed/16504929

Delta9-tetrahydrocannabinol-induced apoptosis in Jurkat leukemia T cells is regulated by translocation of Bad to mitochondria.

Molecular Cancer Research.
Jia W, Hegde VL, Singh NP, Sisco D,
Grant S, Nagarkatti M, Nagarkatti PS.
Department of Pharmacology and Toxicology, Medical College of Virginia Campus, Virginia Commonwealth University, Richmond, USA.

Abstract

Plant-derived cannabinoids, including Delta9-tetrahydrocannabinol (THC), induce apopto-sis in leukemic cells, although the precise mechanism remains unclear. In the current study, we investigated the effect of THC on the upstream and downstream events that modulate the extracellular signal-regulated kinase (ERK) module of mitogen-activated protein kinase pathways primarily in human Jurkat leukemia T cells. The data showed that THC down-regulated Raf-1/mitogen-activated protein kinase/ERK kinase (MEK)/ERK/RSK pathway leading to translocation of Bad to mitochondria. THC also decreased the phospho-rylation of Akt. However, no significant association of Bad translocation with phosphati-dylinositol 3-kinase/Akt and protein kinase A signaling pathways was noted when treated cells were examined in relation to phosphorylation status of Bad by Western blot and localization of Bad to mitochondria by confocal analysis. Furthermore, THC treatment decreased the Bad phosphorylation at Ser(112) but failed to alter the level of phospho-Bad on site Ser(136) that has been reported to be associated with phosphatidylinositol 3-kinase/Akt signal pathway. Jurkat cells expressing a constitutively active MEK construct were found to be resistant to THC-mediated apoptosis and failed to exhibit decreased phospho-Bad on Ser(112) as well as Bad translocation to mitochondria. Finally, use of Bad small interfering RNA reduced the expression of Bad in Jurkat cells leading to increased resistance to THC-mediated apoptosis. Together, these data suggested that Raf 1/MEK/ERK/RSK-mediated Bad translocation played a critical role in THC-induced apoptosis in Jurkat cells.

PubMed Link: https://www.ncbi.nlm.nih.gov/pubmed/16908594

"Numerous studies have shown that THC can modulate the functions of immune cells (7). More recently, we reported that the immunosuppressive property of THC can be attributed, at least in part, to its ability to induce apoptosis in T cells and dendritic cells through ligation of CB2 receptors and that the latter was regulated by activation of nuclear factor-κB (8), recruiting both intrinsic and extrinsic pathways of apoptosis. Interestingly, we also found that THC and other cannabinoids could induce apoptosis in transformed murine and human T cells (9), including primary acute lymphoblastic human leukemia cells, and furthermore that the treatment of mice bearing a T-cell leukemia with THC could cure ~25% of the mice (10). These findings are consistent with studies showing that THC and other cannabinoids can induce apoptosis in a variety of tumor cell lines, thereby raising the possibility of the use of cannabinoids as novel anticancer agents (11). The precise mechanism through which cannabinoids induce apoptosis is under active investigation and may vary based on cell type."

Complete Study Links:

http://mcr.aacrjournals.org/content/4/8/549.long
http://mcr.aacrjournals.org/content/4/8/549.full-text.pdf

Distinctive Pattern of Cannabinoid Receptor Type II (CB2) Expression in Adult and Pediatric Brain Tumors
Brain Research
A Ellert-Miklaszewska et al.

Abstract

The efficacy of cannabinoids against high-grade glioma in animal models, mediated by two specific receptors, CB1 and CB2, raised promises for targeted treatment of the most frequent and malignant primary brain tumors. Unlike the abundantly expressed CB1, the CB2 receptor shows a restricted distribution in normal brain. Although brain tumors constitute the second most common malignancy in children and the prevalence of histological types of brain tumors vary significantly between the adult and pediatric populations, cannabinoid receptor expression in pediatric tumors remains unknown. In the present study, we compared the expression of the CB2 receptor in paraffin-embedded sections from primary brain tumors of adult and pediatric patients. Most glioblastomas expressed very high levels of CB2 receptors and the expression correlated with tumor grade. Interestingly, some benign pediatric astrocytic tumors, such as subependymal giant cell astrocytoma (SEGA), which may occasionally cause mortality owing to progressive growth, also displayed high CB2 immunoreactivity. The high levels of CB2 expression would predestine those tumors to be vulnerable to cannabinoid treatment. In contrast, all examined cases of embryonal tumors (medulloblastoma and S-PNET), the most frequently diagnosed malignant brain tumors in childhood, showed no or trace CB2 immunoreactivity. Our results suggest that the CB2 receptor expression depends primarily on the histopathological origin of the brain tumor cells and differentiation state, reflecting the tumor grade.

PubMed Link: https://www.ncbi.nlm.nih.gov/labs/articles/17239827/

Delta9-tetrahydrocannabinol inhibits cell cycle progression in human breast cancer cells through Cdc2 regulation.

Cancer Research.

Caffarel MM, Sarrió D, Palacios J, Guzmán M, Sánchez C.
Department of Biochemistry and Molecular Biology I, School of Biology,
Complutense University, Madrid, Spain.

Abstract

It has been proposed that cannabinoids are involved in the control of cell fate. Thus, these compounds can modulate proliferation, differentiation, and survival in different manners depending on the cell type and its physiopathologic context. However, little is known about the effect of cannabinoids on the cell cycle, the main process controlling cell fate. Here, we show that Delta(9)-tetrahydrocannabinol (THC), through activation of CB(2) cannabinoid receptors, reduces human breast cancer cell proliferation by blocking the progression of the cell cycle and by inducing apoptosis. In particular, THC arrests cells in G(2)-M via down-regulation of Cdc2, as suggested by the decreased sensitivity to THC acquired by Cdc2-overexpressing cells. Of interest, the proliferation pattern of normal human mammary epithelial cells was much less affected by THC. We also analyzed by real-time quantitative PCR the expression of CB(1) and CB(2) cannabinoid receptors in a series of human breast tumor and nontumor samples. We found a correlation between CB(2) expression and histologic grade of the tumors. There was also an association between CB(2) expression and other markers of prognostic and predictive value, such as estrogen receptor, progesterone receptor, and ERBB2/HER-2 oncogene. Importantly, no significant CB(2) expression was detected in nontumor breast tissue. Taken together, these data might set the bases for a cannabinoid therapy for the management of breast cancer.

PubMed Link: https://www.ncbi.nlm.nih.gov/pubmed/16818634

FROM FULL TEXT:

"There are very few critical decisions that cells must take during their lifetime. Basically, these are whether to proliferate, differentiate, or die. A tight regulation of the cell cycle is crucial to control all these decisions, and its deregulation has devastating consequences, such as cancer (1). It has been proposed that cannabinoids, the active components of Cannabis sativa, play a role in the control of the aforementioned decisions. For example, they can modulate survival, proliferation, and differentiation depending on the cell type and its physiopathologic context (2, 3). Among the 70 cannabinoids synthesized by C. sativa, D9-tetrahydrocannabinol (THC) is the most important in terms of potency and abundance (4). THC exerts a wide variety of biological effects by mimicking endogenous compounds, the endocannabinoids anandamide and 2-arachidonoylglycerol, which activate specific cannabinoid receptors."

Complete Study Links:

http://cancerres.aacrjournals.org/content/66/13/6615
http://cancerres.aacrjournals.org/content/66/13/6615.full-text.pdf

Cannabinoids induce apoptosis of pancreatic tumor cells via endoplasmic reticulum stress-related genes.
Cancer Research.

Carracedo A, Gironella M, Lorente M, Garcia S,
Guzmán M, Velasco G, Iovanna JL.
Department of Biochemistry and Molecular Biology I, School of Biology,
Complutense University, c/José Antonio Novais, Madrid, Spain.

Abstract
Pancreatic adenocarcinomas are among the most malignant forms of cancer and, therefore, it is of especial interest to set new strategies aimed at improving the prognostic of this deadly disease. The present study was undertaken to investigate the action of cannabinoids, a new family of potential antitumoral agents, in pancreatic cancer. We show that cannabinoid receptors are expressed in human pancreatic tumor cell lines and tumor biopsies at much higher levels than in normal pancreatic tissue. Studies conducted with MiaPaCa2 and Panc1 cell lines showed that cannabinoid administration (a) induced apoptosis, (b) increased ceramide levels, and (c) up-regulated mRNA levels of the stress protein p8. These effects were prevented by blockade of the CB(2) cannabinoid receptor or by pharmacologic inhibition of ceramide synthesis de novo. Knockdown experiments using selective small interfering RNAs showed the involvement of p8 via its downstream endoplasmic reticulum stress-related targets activating transcription factor 4 (ATF-4) and TRB3 in Delta(9)-tetrahydrocannabinol-induced apoptosis. Cannabinoids also reduced the growth of tumor cells in two animal models of pancreatic cancer. In addition, cannabinoid treatment inhibited the spreading of pancreatic tumor cells. Moreover, cannabinoid administration selectively increased apoptosis and TRB3 expression in pancreatic tumor cells but not in normal tissue. In conclusion, results presented here show that cannabinoids lead to apoptosis of pancreatic tumor cells via a CB(2) receptor and de novo synthesized ceramide-dependent up-regulation of p8 and the endoplasmic reticulum stress-related genes ATF-4 and TRB3. These findings may contribute to set the basis for a new therapeutic approach for the treatment of pancreatic cancer.

PubMed Link: https://www.ncbi.nlm.nih.gov/pubmed/16818650

FROM FULL TEXT:

"Pancreatic cancer is one of the most malignant and aggressive forms of cancer (1). With an incidence of 10/10,000 for men and 7/10,000 for women, it represents the fourth most common deathcausing cancer in the United States (2) and the fifth in the Western world overall (3). About 95% of pancreatic cancers cases are ductal adenocarcinomas. The anatomic localization of the pancreas and the nonspecific nature of the symptoms result in a complex and delayed diagnosis. Therefore, at the time of detection, 85% of patients show metastasic infiltrations in proximal lymphatic nodes, liver, or lungs, and only 15% to 20% of the tumors are typically found resectable (1). In addition, <20% of the operated patients survive up to 5 years. Treatment of unresectable tumors is currently based on administration of fluorouracil chemoradiation for locally advanced tumors and gemcitabine chemotherapy for metastatic disease (1). However, despite maximal optimization of these therapies, the median survival for the affected patients remains 1 year. It is therefore of especial interest to set new therapeutic strategies aimed at improving the prognostic of this deadly disease. The hemp plant Cannabis sativa produces f70 unique compounds known as cannabinoids, of which D9-tetrahydrocannabinol (THC) is the most important owing to its high potency and abundance in cannabis (4).

Results

Activation of the CB2 cannabinoid receptor induces apoptosis of pancreatic tumor cells in vitro. We investigated the effect of cannabinoids on pancreatic tumor cells...Incubation with THC led to a dose-dependent decrease in cell viability in the four lines tested (Fig. 2A). Because cells exhibited a different sensitivity to THC treatment, we chose MiaPaCa2 as the most sensitive line and Panc1 as a less sensitive line to confirm the involvement of cannabinoid receptors in THC antiproliferative action. Incubation with the CB2-selective antagonist SR144528, but not with the CB1-selective antagonist SR141716, prevented THCinduced loss of cell viability in both lines (Fig. 2B and C). Likewise, in MiaPaca2 and Panc1 cells, THC led to caspase-3 activation, a characteristic of apoptotic cell death, and preincubation with SR144528 abrogated this effect (Fig. 2D and E)."

Complete Study Links:

http://cancerres.aacrjournals.org/content/66/13/6748.long
http://cancerres.aacrjournals.org/content/66/13/6748.full-text.pdf

A pilot clinical study of Delta9-tetrahydrocannabinol in patients with recurrent glioblastoma multiforme.
British Journal of Cancer.

Guzmán M, Duarte MJ, Blázquez C, Ravina J, Rosa MC, Galve-Roperh I, Sánchez C, Velasco G, González-Feria L.
Department of Biochemistry and Molecular Biology I, School of Biology, Complutense University, Madrid, Spain.

Abstract
Delta(9)-Tetrahydrocannabinol (THC) and other cannabinoids inhibit tumour growth and angiogenesis in animal models, so their potential application as antitumoral drugs has been suggested. However, the antitumoral effect of cannabinoids has never been tested in humans. Here we report the first clinical study aimed at assessing cannabinoid antitumoral action, specifically a pilot phase I trial in which nine patients with recurrent glioblastoma multiforme were administered THC intratumoraly. The patients had previously failed standard therapy (surgery and radiotherapy) and had clear evidence of tumour progression. The primary end point of the study was to determine the safety of intracranial THC administration. We also evaluated THC action on the length of survival and various tumour-cell parameters. A dose escalation regimen for THC administration was assessed. Cannabinoid delivery was safe and could be achieved without overt psychoactive effects. Median survival of the cohort from the beginning of cannabinoid administration was 24 weeks (95% confidence interval: 15-33). Delta(9)-Tetrahydrocannabinol inhibited tumour-cell proliferation in vitro and decreased tumour-cell Ki67 immunostaining when adminis-

tered to two patients. The fair safety profile of THC, together with its possible antiproliferative action on tumour cells reported here and in other studies, may set the basis for future trials aimed at evaluating the potential antitumoral activity of cannabinoids.

PubMed Link: https://www.ncbi.nlm.nih.gov/pubmed/16804518

FROM FULL TEXT:

"One of the most devastating forms of cancer is glioblastoma multiforme (grade IV astrocytoma), the most frequent class of malignant primary brain tumours. Current standard therapeutic strategies for the treatment of glioblastoma multiforme (surgical resection and focal radiotherapy) are only palliative, and, as a consequence, survival after diagnosis is normally 6–12 months (Afra et al, 2002; Kleihues et al, 2002; Lonardi et al, 2005). A large number of chemotherapeutic agents (e.g. alkylating agents such as temozolomide and nitrosoureas such as carmustine) have also been tested, but no remarkable improvement on patient survival has been achieved as yet (Afra et al, 2002; Lonardi et al, 2005; Reardon et al, 2006). Likewise, although dendritic cell- and peptide-based immunotherapy strategies appear promising as a safe approach to induce an antitumour immune response (Yamanaka, 2006), no immunotherapy or gene therapy trial performed to date has been significantly successful. It is therefore essential to develop new therapeutic strategies for the management of glioblastoma multiforme to obtain significant clinical results. We have previously shown that cannabinoids inhibit the growth (Galve-Roperh et al, 2000; Sánchez et al, 2001) and angiogenesis (Blázquez et al, 2003, 2004) of gliomas in animal models. Remarkably, this antiproliferative effect seems to be selective for brain-tumour cells as the survival of normal brain cells (astrocytes (Gómez del Pulgar et al, 2002), oligodendrocytes (Molina-Holgado et al, 2002) and neurons (Mechoulam et al, 2002)) is unaffected or even favoured by cannabinoid challenge. On the basis of these preclinical findings, we have conducted a pilot clinical study aimed at assessing cannabinoid antitumoral action in patients with recurrent glioblastoma multiforme...Here we report the first clinical study aimed at evaluating cannabinoid antitumoral action. Owing to obvious ethical and legal reasons, this pilot study was conducted in a cohort of terminal patients harbouring actively growing recurrent tumours. Although the use of cannabinoids in medicine may be limited by their well-known psychotropic effects, it is generally believed that cannabinoids display a fair drug safety profile and that their potential adverse effects are within the range of those accepted for other medications, especially in cancer treatment (Guzmán, 2003; Hall et al, 2005; Iversen, 2005). In line with this idea, THC delivery in our study was safe and could be achieved without overt psychoactive effects. As the possible antitumoral action of nabilone has never been evaluated in preclinical trials, THC was the unique cannabinoid receptor agonist available for the present human study. Nonetheless, most likely THC is not the most appropriate cannabinoid agonist for future antitumoral strategies owing to its high hydrophobicity, relatively weak agonistic potency and ability to elicit CB1-mediated psychoactivity. ...In view of the fair safety profile of THC, together with its possible antiproliferative action on tumour cells reported here and in other studies (Guzmán, 2003), it would be desirable that additional trials – on this and other types of tumours – were run to determine whether cannabinoids – as single drugs or in combination with established antitumoral drugs – could be used, other than for their palliative effects, to inhibit tumour growth. In particular, our next goal is to evaluate the efficacy of THC in patients with newly diagnosed gliobastoma multiforme."

Complete Study Links:

http://www.nature.com/bjc/journal/v95/n2/full/6603236a.html
http://www.nature.com/bjc/journal/v95/n2/pdf/6603236a.pdf

Cannabinoid derivatives induce cell death in pancreatic MIA PaCa-2 cells via a receptor-independent mechanism.

FEBS Letters.

Fogli S, Nieri P, Chicca A, Adinolfi B, Mariotti V, Iacopetti P, Breschi MC, Pellegrini S.
Department of Psychiatry, University of Pisa, Pisa, PI, Italy.

Abstract

Cannabinoids (CBs) are implicated in the control of cell survival in different types of tumors, but little is known about the role of CB system in pancreatic cancer. Herein, we investigated the in vitro antitumor activity of CBs and the potential role of their receptors in human pancreatic cancer cells MIA PaCa-2. Characterization tools used for this study included growth inhibition/cell viability analyses, caspase 3/7 induction, DNA fragmentation, microarray analysis and combination index-isobologram method. Our results demonstrate that CBs produce a significant cytotoxic effect via a receptor-independent mechanism. The CB1 antagonist N-(piperidin-1-1yl)-5-(4-iodophenyl)-1-(2,4-dichlorophenyl)-4-methyl-1H-pyrazole-3-carboxamide (AM251) was the most active compound with an IC50 of 8.6 +/- 1.3 microM after 72 h. AM251 induces apoptosis, causes transcriptional changes of genes in janus kinase/signal transducers and activators of transcription signaling network and synergistically interacts with the pyrimidine analogue, 5-fluorouracil. These findings exclude the involvement of CB receptors in the regulation of MIA PaCa-2 cell growth and put AM251 forward as a candidate for the development of novel compounds worthy to be tested in this type of neoplasia.

PubMed Link: https://www.ncbi.nlm.nih.gov/pubmed/16500647

Overexpression of cannabinoid receptors CB1 and CB2 correlates with improved prognosis of patients with hepatocellular carcinoma.

Cancer Genetics and Cytogenetics.

Xu X, Liu Y, Huang S, Liu G, Xie C, Zhou J, Fan W,
Li Q, Wang Q, Zhong D, Miao X.
Department of Surgery, Xiangya 2nd Hospital, Central South University,
Changsha City, Hunan Province, China.

Abstract
CB1 and CB2 are multifunctional cannabinoid-specific receptors considered to be involved in inhibition of tumor development. To elucidate their roles in hepatocarcinogenesis, we analyzed the expression of these receptors in tumor and matched nontumorous tissues of human hepatocellular carcinoma (HCC) samples. In situ hybridization analysis showed overexpression of CB1 mRNAs in 8 of 13 (62%) HCC samples, and of CB2 mRNAs in 7 of 13 (54%). Immunohistochemical analysis of 64 HCC samples showed the expression of CB1 and CB2 receptors to increase from normal liver to chronic hepatitis to cirrhosis. Marked expression of CB1 and CB2 receptors was noted in the majority of cirrhotic liver samples (86 and 78%, respectively). In HCC, high expression of CB1 and CB2 receptors was observed in 29 (45%) and 33 (52%) cases, respectively. Clinicopathological evaluation indicated a significant correlation between CB1 and CB2 expression and two clinicopathological parameters such as the histopathological differentiation ($P = 0.021$ and 0.001, respectively), portal vein invasion ($P = 0.015$ and 0.004, respectively). Univariate analysis indicated that disease-free survival was significantly better in HCC patients with high versus those with low CB1 and CB2 expression levels ($P = 0.010$ and 0.037, respectively). Our results indicate that CB1 and CB2 have potential as prognostic indicators and suggest possible beneficial effects of cannabinoids on prognosis of patients with HCC.

PubMed Link: https://www.ncbi.nlm.nih.gov/pubmed/17074588

Cannabinoid receptors as novel targets for the treatment of melanoma.

Federation of American Societies For Experimental Biology

Blázquez C, Carracedo A, Barrado L, Real PJ, Fernández-Luna JL,
Velasco G, Malumbres M, Guzmán M.
Department of Biochemistry and Molecular Biology I, School of Biology,
Complutense University, Madrid, Spain.

Abstract
Melanoma causes the greatest number of skin cancer-related deaths worldwide. Despite intensive research, prevention and early detection are the only effective measures against melanoma, so new therapeutic strategies are necessary for the management of this devastating disease. Here, we evaluated the efficacy of cannabinoid receptor agonists, a new family of potential antitumoral compounds, at skin melanoma. Human melanomas and

melanoma cell lines express CB1 and CB2 cannabinoid receptors. Activation of these receptors decreased growth, proliferation, angiogenesis and metastasis, and increased apoptosis, of melanomas in mice. Cannabinoid antimelanoma activity was independent of the immune status of the animal, could be achieved without overt psychoactive effects and was selective for melanoma cells vs. normal melanocytes. Cannabinoid antiproliferative action on melanoma cells was due, at least in part, to cell cycle arrest at the G1-S transition via inhibition of the prosurvival protein Akt and hypophosphorylation of the pRb retinoblastoma protein tumor suppressor. These findings may contribute to the design of new chemotherapeutic strategies for the management of melanoma.

PubMed Link: https://www.ncbi.nlm.nih.gov/pubmed/17065222

FROM FULL TEXT:

"Melanoma causes the greatest number of skin cancer-related deaths both in the USA (1) and worldwide(2). In 2005, an estimated 59,600 Americans were diagnosed with this cancer and 7,800 died of it (1, 3)... Despite intensive research, no effective therapies exist for advanced melanoma....cannabinoids are potential antitumoral agents owing to their ability to inhibit the growth and angiogenesis of various types of tumor xenografts in animal models (11, 13–15). Cannabinoids display a fair drug safety profile in both animals and humans and do not produce the generalized cytotoxic effects of conventional chemotherapies (11, 16–18). In this context, we have recently run a pilot clinical trial aimed at investigating the effect of THC administration on the growth of recurrent glioblastoma multiforme....

Activation of cannabinoid receptors decreases melanoma cell proliferation, at least in part, via inhibition of Akt, a key element of a major prosurvival pathway that is deregulated in many types of tumors, including melanoma (5, 36, 37).... Although the use of cannabinoids in medicine is limited by their psychotropic effects, these compounds display a fair drug safety profile; their potential adverse effects are within the range of those accepted for other medications—especially in cancer treatment—and their psychoactive effects tend to disappear with tolerance on continuous use (11, 12). Nonetheless, it is obvious that cannabinoid based therapies devoid of side effects would be desirable. As the unwanted effects of cannabinoids are mediated largely or entirely by CB1 receptors within the brain, the most conceivable possibility would be to use cannabinoids that selectively target CB2 receptors. Although under certain circumstances CB2 receptor activation in immune cells may blunt host antitumor activity, as discussed elsewhere (11, 43), this may be evident only in particular experimental conditions, and indeed most of the data obtained so far from animal models of cancer have demonstrated a tumor growth-inhibiting action of cannabinoids (11). In this context, here, we show that CB2 receptor activation is functional in curbing melanoma cell growth in vitro and in vivo, the latter under conditions previously observed to produce no overt signs of psychoactivity (43)."

Complete Study Link:

http://bbml.ucm.es/cannabis/archivos/publicaciones/FASEB_J06_20_263 3_2635.pdf

Antitumor activity of plant cannabinoids with emphasis on the effect of cannabidiol on human breast carcinoma.

The Journal of Pharmacology and Experimental Theraputics.

Ligresti A, Moriello AS, Starowicz K, Matias I, Pisanti S, De Petrocellis L, Laezza C, Portella G, Bifulco M, Di Marzo V.
Istituto di Chimica Biomolecolare, Consiglio Nazionale delle Ricerche Pozzuoli, Italy.

Abstract

Delta(9)-Tetrahydrocannabinol (THC) exhibits antitumor effects on various cancer cell types, but its use in chemotherapy is limited by its psychotropic activity. We investigated the antitumor activities of other plant cannabinoids, i.e., cannabidiol, cannabigerol, cannabichromene, cannabidiol acid and THC acid, and assessed whether there is any advantage in using Cannabis extracts (enriched in either cannabidiol or THC) over pure cannabinoids. Results obtained in a panel of tumor cell lines clearly indicate that, of the five natural compounds tested, cannabidiol is the most potent inhibitor of cancer cell growth (IC(50) between 6.0 and 10.6 microM), with significantly lower potency in noncancer cells. The cannabidiol-rich extract was equipotent to cannabidiol, whereas cannabigerol and cannabichromene followed in the rank of potency. Both cannabidiol and the cannabidiol-rich extract inhibited the growth of xenograft tumors obtained by s.c. injection into athymic mice of human MDA-MB-231 breast carcinoma or rat v-K-ras-transformed thyroid epithelial cells and reduced lung metastases deriving from intrapaw injection of MDA-MB-231 cells. Judging from several experiments on its possible cellular and molecular mechanisms of action, we propose that cannabidiol lacks a unique mode of action in the cell lines investigated. At least for MDA-MB-231 cells, however, our experiments indicate that cannabidiol effect is due to its capability of inducing apoptosis via: direct or indirect activation of cannabinoid CB(2) and vanilloid transient receptor potential vanilloid type-1 receptors and cannabinoid/vanilloid receptor-independent elevation of intracellular Ca(2+) and reactive oxygen species. Our data support the further testing of cannabidiol and cannabidiol-rich extracts for the potential treatment of cancer.

PubMed Link: https://www.ncbi.nlm.nih.gov/pubmed/16728591

FROM FULL TEXT:

"The aim of this study was to identify natural cannabinoids with antitumor activities at least similar to those of THC and devoid of the potential central effects of this compound. Given that the efficacy of cannabinoids as antitumoral agents appears to be strictly correlated to the cell type under investigation, we screened a panel of plant cannabinoids in a wide range of tumoral cell lines distinct in origin and typology. We found that, surprisingly, cannabidiol acted as a more potent inhibitor of cancer cell growth than THC and that cannabigerol and cannabichromene usually followed cannabidiol in the rank of potency. The cell growth-inhibitory effect of cannabidiol depended on its chemical structure since the addition of a carboxylic acid group (as in cannabidiol acid) dramatically reduced its activity. This is unlikely due to simple modification of the lipophilicity of the compound and subsequent decrease of its capability to penetrate the cell membrane since THC-A was often more efficacious than THC. We also found that the cannabidiol-rich Cannabis extract was as potent as pure cannabidiol in most cases or even more potent in some cell lines. These results suggest the use in cancer therapy for cannabidiol, a compound lacking the psychotropic effects typical of THC. Indeed, the efficacy of cannabidiol and of the cannabidiol-rich extract were confirmed in vivo in two different models of xenograft tumors obtained by inoculation in athymic mice of either v-K-ras-transformed thyroid epithelial cells or of the highly invasive MDA-MB-231 breast cancer cells. Furthermore, cannabidiol and the cannabidiolrich extract also inhibited the formation of lung metastases subsequent to inoculation of MDA-MB-231 cells, in agreement with the inhibitory actions on cancer cell migration previously described for this compound (Vaccani et al., 2005).

Complete Study Links:
http://jpet.aspetjournals.org/content/318/3/1375
http://jpet.aspetjournals.org/content/jpet/318/3/1375.full.pdf

2007

Endocannabinoids as emerging suppressors of angiogenesis and tumor invasion (review).
Oncology Reports.

Bifulco M, Laezza C, Gazzerro P, Pentimalli F.
Dipartimento di Scienze Farmaceutiche, Università degli Studi di Salerno, Fisciano (SA), Italy.

Abstract

The medicinal properties of extracts from the hemp plant Cannabis sativa have been known for centuries but only in the 90s membrane receptors for the Cannabis major principle were discovered in mammalian cells. Later on the endogenous ligands for the cannabinoid receptors were identified and the term 'endocannabinoid system' was coined to indicate the complex signaling system of cannabinoid receptors, endogenous ligands and the enzymes responsible for their biosynthesis and inactivation. The 'endocannabinoid system' is involved in a broad range of functions and in a growing number of pathological conditions. There is increasing evidence that endocannabinoids are able to inhibit cancer cell growth in culture as well as in animal models. Most work has focused on the role of endocannabinoids in regulating tumor cell growth and apoptosis and ongoing research is addressed to further dissect the precise mechanisms of cannabinoid antitumor action. However, endocannabinoids are now emerging as suppressors of angiogenesis and tumor spreading since they have been reported to inhibit angiogenesis, cell migration and metastasis in different types of cancer, pointing to a potential role of the endocannabinoid system as a target for a therapeutic approach of such malignant diseases. The potential use of cannabinoids to retard tumor growth and spreading is even more appealing considering that they show a good safety profile, regarding toxicity, and are already used in cancer patients as palliatives to stimulate appetite and to prevent devastating effects such as nausea, vomiting and pain.

PubMed Link: https://www.ncbi.nlm.nih.gov/pubmed/17342320

Cannabinoids and gliomas.
Molecular Neurobiology.

Velasco G, Carracedo A, Blázquez C, Lorente M, Aguado T, Haro A, Sánchez C, Galve-Roperh I, Guzmán M.
Department of Biochemistry and Molecular Biology I, School of Biology, Complutense University, Madrid, Spain.

Abstract

   Cannabinoids, the active components of Cannabis sativa L., act in the body by mimicking endogenous substances--the endocannabinoids--that activate specific cell surface receptors. Cannabinoids exert various palliative effects in cancer patients. In addition, cannabinoids inhibit the growth of different types of tumor cells, including glioma cells, in laboratory animals. They do so by modulating key cell signaling pathways, mostly the endoplasmic reticulum stress response, thereby inducing antitumoral actions such as the apoptotic death of tumor cells and the inhibition of tumor angiogenesis. Of interest, cannabinoids seem to be selective antitumoral compounds, as they kill glioma cells, but not their non-transformed astroglial counterparts. On the basis of these preclinical findings, a pilot clinical study of Delta(9)-tetrahydrocannabinol (THC) in patients with recurrent glioblastoma multiforme has been recently run. The good safety profile of THC, together with its possible growth-inhibiting action on tumor cells, justifies the setting up of future trials aimed at evaluating the potential antitumoral activity of cannabinoids.

PubMed Link: https://www.ncbi.nlm.nih.gov/pubmed/17952650

The endocannabinoid system in cancer-potential therapeutic target?
Seminars in Cancer Biology.

Flygare J, Sander B.
Department of Laboratory Medicine, Divison of Pathology, Karolinska Institutet and Karolinska University Hospital Huddinge, Stockholm, Sweden.

Abstract

Endogenous arachidonic acid metabolites with properties similar to compounds of Cannabis sativa Linnaeus, the so-called endocannabinoids, have effects on various types of cancer. Although endocannabinoids and synthetic cannabinoids may have pro-proliferative effects, predominantly inhibitory effects on tumor growth, angiogenesis, migration and metastasis have been described. Remarkably, these effects may be selective for the cancer cells, while normal cells and tissues are spared. Such apparent tumor cell selectivity makes the endocannabinoid system an attractive potential target for cancer therapy. In this review we discuss various means by which the endocannabinoid system may be targeted in cancer and the current knowledge considering the regulation of the endocannabinoid system in malignancy.

PubMed Link: https://www.ncbi.nlm.nih.gov/pubmed/18249558

FROM FULL TEXT:
"The natural plant cannabinoid, ^-9-tetrahydrocannabinol (THC) was recognized as a potential anti-cancer agent already in 1975 [12]. However, it was not until the last 10–15 years that further studies in this area were carried out. Since then, there has been a great effort to investigate the therapeutic potentialof cannabinoids in various types of cancer [13] and a first human clinical study has been performed [14]. Cannabinoids have been found to control cell growth and death in many cancer types but the mechanisms underlying the antitumor effects may vary and are sometimes cell type specific. Cannabinoids have been reported to cause heterogeneous effects in tumor cells, such as cell cycle alterations resulting in growth arrest, induction of apoptosis, anti-angiogenic activity and reduced migration. In some instances pro-proliferative effects of cannabinoids have been reported."

Complete Study Link:
http://theroc.us/images/The%20endocannabinoid%20system%20in%20cancer-%20Potential%20therapeutic%20target.pdf

Cannabinoid receptor agonists are mitochondrial inhibitors: a unified hypothesis of how cannabinoids modulate mitochondrial function and induce cell death.

Biochememical and Biophysical Research Communications.

Athanasiou A, Clarke AB, Turner AE, Kumaran NM, Vakilpour S, Smith PA, Bagiokou D, Bradshaw TD, Westwell AD, Fang L, Lobo DN, Constantinescu CS, Calabrese V, Loesch A, Alexander SP, Clothier RH, Kendall DA, Bates TE.

School of Biomedical Sciences, University of Nottingham, Queen's Medical Centre, Nottingham, UK.

Abstract

Time-lapse microscopy of human lung cancer (H460) cells showed that the endogenous cannabinoid anandamide (AEA), the phyto-cannabinoid Delta-9-tetrahydrocannabinol (THC) and a synthetic cannabinoid HU 210 all caused morphological changes characteristic of apoptosis. Janus green assays of H460 cell viability showed that AEA and THC caused significant increases in OD 595 nm at lower concentrations (10-50 microM) and

115

significant decreases at 100 microM, whilst HU 210 caused significant decreases at all concentrations. In rat heart mitochondria, all three ligands caused significant decreases in oxygen consumption and mitochondrial membrane potential. THC and HU 210 caused significant increases in mitochondrial hydrogen peroxide production, whereas AEA was without significant effect. All three ligands induced biphasic changes in either mitochondrial complex I activity and/or mitochondrial complex II-III activity. These data demonstrate that AEA, THC, and HU 210 are all able to cause changes in integrated mitochondrial function, directly, in the absence of cannabinoid receptors.

PubMed Link: https://www.ncbi.nlm.nih.gov/pubmed/17931597

Cannabinoids induce glioma stem-like cell differentiation and inhibit gliomagenesis.

Journal of Biological Chemistry.

Aguado T, Carracedo A, Julien B, Velasco G, Milman G, Mechoulam R, Alvarez L, Guzmán M, Galve-Roperh I.

Department of Biochemistry and Molecular Biology I, School of Biology, Complutense University, Madrid, Spain.

Abstract

Glioma stem-like cells constitute one of the potential origins of gliomas, and therefore, their elimination is an essential factor for the development of efficient therapeutic strategies. Cannabinoids are known to exert an antitumoral action on gliomas that relies on at least two mechanisms: induction of apoptosis of transformed cells and inhibition of tumor angiogenesis. However, whether cannabinoids target human glioma stem cells and their potential impact in gliomagenesis are unknown. Here, we show that glioma stem-like cells derived from glioblastoma multiforme biopsies and the glioma cell lines U87MG and U373MG express cannabinoid type 1 (CB(1)) and type 2 (CB(2)) receptors and other elements of the endocannabinoid system. In gene array experiments, CB receptor activation altered the expression of genes involved in the regulation of stem cell proliferation and differentiation. The cannabinoid agonists HU-210 and JWH-133 promoted glial differentiation in a CB receptor-dependent manner as shown by the increased number of S-100beta- and glial fibrillary acidic protein-expressing cells. In parallel, cannabinoids decreased the cell population expressing the neuroepithelial progenitor marker nestin. Moreover, cannabinoid challenge decreased the efficiency of glioma stem-like cells to initiate glioma formation in vivo, a finding that correlated with decreased neurosphere formation and cell proliferation in secondary xenografts. Gliomas derived from cannabinoid-treated cancer stem-like cells were characterized with a panel of neural markers and evidenced a more differentiated phenotype and a concomitant decrease in nestin expression. Overall, our results demonstrate that cannabinoids target glioma stem-like cells, promote their differentiation, and inhibit gliomagenesis, thus giving further support to their potential use in the management of malignant gliomas.

PubMed Link: https://www.ncbi.nlm.nih.gov/pubmed/17202146

FROM FULL TEXT:

"Malignant gliomas remain the most deadly human brain tumors, with poor prognosis despite years of research in antitumoral therapeutic strategies...Among those strategies, cannabinoid-based drugs may represent an alternative to other established chemotherapeutics (12). The discovery of an endogenous cannabinoid system (13), together with the great improvement in our understanding of the signaling mechanisms responsible for cannabinoid actions (12, 13), has fostered the interest in the potential therapeutic applications of cannabinoids (14). Several studies have demonstrated a significant antitumoral action of cannabinoid ligands in animal models (12). Thus, cannabinoid administration to nude mice curbs the growth of different tumors, including gliomas, lung adenocarcinomas, thyroid epitheliomas, lymphomas, and skin carcinomas (12). The antitumoral action on gliomas relies on at least two mechanisms: induction of apoptosis of tumor cells (15, 16) and inhibition of tumor angiogenesis (17)."

Complete Study Links:

http://www.jbc.org/content/282/9/6854.long
http://www.jbc.org/content/282/9/6854.full.pdf

Delta9-Tetrahydrocannabinol inhibits epithelial growth factor-induced lung cancer cell migration in vitro as well as its growth and metastasis in vivo.

Oncogene.

Preet A, Ganju RK, Groopman JE.
Division of Experimental Medicine, Department of Medicine, Beth Israel Deaconess Medical Center, Harvard Medical School, Boston, MA, USA.

Abstract:

"Delta(9)-Tetrahydrocannabinol (THC) is the primary cannabinoid of marijuana and has been shown to either potentiate or inhibit tumor growth, depending on the type of cancer and its pathogenesis. Little is known about the activity of cannabinoids like THC on epidermal growth factor receptor-overexpressing lung cancers, which are often highly aggressive and resistant to chemotherapy. In this study, we characterized the effects of THC on the EGF-induced growth and metastasis of human non-small cell lung cancer using the cell lines A549 and SW-1573 as in vitro models. We found that these cells express the cannabinoid receptors CB(1) and CB(2), known targets for THC action, and that THC inhibited EGF-induced growth, chemotaxis and chemoinvasion. Moreover, signaling studies indicated that THC may act by inhibiting the EGF-induced phosphorylation of ERK1/2, JNK1/2 and AKT. THC also induced the phosphorylation of focal adhesion kinase at tyrosine 397. Additionally, in in vivo studies in severe combined immunodeficient mice, there was significant inhibition of the subcutaneous tumor growth and lung metastasis of A549 cells in THC-treated animals as compared to vehicle-treated controls. Tumor samples from THC-treated animals revealed antiproliferative and antiangiogenic effects of THC. Our study suggests that cannabinoids like THC should be explored as novel therapeutic molecules in controlling the growth and metastasis of certain lung cancers."

PubMed Link: https://www.ncbi.nlm.nih.gov/pubmed/17621270

FROM FULL TEXT:

"We demonstrate for the first time that THC treatment inhibited the EGF-induced migration and invasion of the NSCLC cell lines, A549 and SW-1573. THC also inhibited the EGF-induced proliferation of these cells. Furthermore, we show that these inhibitory effects of THC were correlated with reductions in the EGF-induced phosphorylation of AKT and mitogen-activated protein (MAP) kinases (ERK1/2 and JNK1/2). Both AKT and MAP kinase pathways are known to play an important role in cancer cell migration and invasion (Williams et al.,1993; Bost et al., 1997; Clarke et al., 1998). We then confirmed the inhibitory effects of THC on tumor growth and metastasis in vivo (Guzma´n et al., 2006). These results provide the basis for studying cannabinoids in the treatment of lung cancer."

Complete Study Links:
http://www.nature.com/onc/journal/v27/n3/full/1210641a.html
http://www.nature.com/onc/journal/v27/n3/pdf/1210641a.pdf

The cannabinoid delta(9)-tetrahydrocannabinol inhibits RAS-MAPK and PI3K-AKT survival signalling and induces BAD-mediated apoptosis in colorectal cancer cells.

International Journal of Cancer.
Greenhough A, Patsos HA, Williams AC, Paraskeva C.
Department of Cellular and Molecular Medicine, Cancer Research UK, Colorectal Tumour Biology Group, School of Medical Sciences, University of Bristol, University Walk, Bristol, United Kingdom.

Abstract (edited):
"There is emerging evidence that cannabinoids, especially Delta(9)-tetrahydrocannabinol (THC), may represent novel anticancer agents, due to their ability to regulate signalling pathways critical for cell growth and survival. Here, we report that CB1 and CB2 cannabinoid receptors are expressed in human colorectal adenoma and carcinoma cells, and show for the first time that THC induces apoptosis in colorectal cancer cells. ...These data suggest an important role for CB1 receptors and BAD in the regulation of apoptosis in colorectal cancer cells. The use of THC, or selective targeting of the CB1 receptor, may represent a novel strategy for colorectal cancer therapy."

PubMed Link: https://www.ncbi.nlm.nih.gov/pubmed/17583570

Cannabinoids in pancreatic cancer: correlation with survival and pain.
International Journal of Cancer

Michalski CW, Oti FE, Erkan M, Sauliunaite D, Bergmann F, Pacher P, Batkai S, Müller MW, Giese NA, Friess H, Kleeff J.
Department of General Surgery, Technische Universität Munich, Munich, Germany.

Abstract (edited)
"Cannabinoids exert antiproliferative properties in a variety of malignant tumors, including pancreatic ductal adenocarcinoma (PDAC)....There was a significant relationship between low CB1 receptor immunoreactivity or mRNA expression levels ($p = 0.0011$ and $p = 0.026$, respectively), or high FAAH and MGLL cancer cell immunoreactivity ($p = 0.036$ and $p = 0.017$, respectively) and longer survival of PDAC patients. These results are underlined by a significant correlation of high pain scores and increased survival ($p = 0.0343$). CB2 receptor immunoreactivity, CB2 receptor, FAAH and MGLL mRNA expression levels did not correlate with survival. Therefore, changes in the levels of endocannabinoid metabolizing enzymes and cannabinoid receptors on pancreatic cancer cells may affect prognosis and pain status of PDAC patients."

PubMed Link: https://www.ncbi.nlm.nih.gov/pubmed/17943729

Complete Study Links:
http://onlinelibrary.wiley.com/doi/10.1002/ijc.23114/full
http://onlinelibrary.wiley.com/doi/10.1002/ijc.23114/pdf

Increased endocannabinoid levels reduce the development of precancerous lesions in the mouse colon.
Journal of Molecular Medicine

Izzo AA, Aviello G, Petrosino S, Orlando P, Marsicano G, Lutz B, Borrelli F, Capasso R, Nigam S, Capasso F, Di Marzo V;
Endocannabinoid Research Group.
Department of Experimental Pharmacology, University of Naples Federico II, Naples, Italy.

Abstract
Colorectal cancer is an increasingly important cause of death in Western countries. Endocannabinoids inhibit colorectal carcinoma cell proliferation in vitro. In this paper, we investigated the involvement of endocannabinoids on the formation of aberrant crypt foci (ACF, earliest preneoplastic lesions) in the colon mouse in vivo. ACF were induced by azoxymethane (AOM); fatty acid amide hydrolase (FAAH) and cannabinoid receptor messenger ribonucleic acid (mRNA) levels were analyzed by the quantitative reverse transcription polymerase chain reaction (RT-PCR); endocannabinoid levels were measured by liquid chromatography-mass spectrometry; caspase-3 and caspase-9 expressions were

measured by Western blot analysis. Colonic ACF formation after AOM administration was associated with increased levels of 2-arachidonoylglycerol (with no changes in FAAH and cannabinoid receptor mRNA levels) and reduction in cleaved caspase-3 and caspase-9 expression. The FAAH inhibitor N-arachidonoylserotonin increased colon endocannabinoid levels, reduced ACF formation, and partially normalized cleaved caspase-3 (but not caspase-9) expression. Notably, N-arachidonoylserotonin completely prevented the formation of ACF with four or more crypts, which have been show to be best correlated with final tumor incidence. The effect of N-arachidonoylserotonin on ACF formation was mimicked by the cannabinoid receptor agonist HU-210. No differences in ACF formation were observed between CB(1) receptor-deficient and wild-type mice. It is concluded that pharmacological enhancement of endocannabinoid levels (through inhibition of endocannabinoid hydrolysis) reduces the development of precancerous lesions in the mouse colon. The protective effect appears to involve caspase-3 (but not caspase-9) activation.

PubMed Link: https://www.ncbi.nlm.nih.gov/pubmed/17823781

FROM FULL TEXT:

"Colon cancer remains a leading cause of death because of cancer in the Western countries; the cumulative lifetime risk of developing colorectal cancer is approximately 5–6% [1]. Development of colon cancer is a multistep process involving a series of pathological alterations ranging from discrete microscopic mucosal lesions, like aberrant crypt foci (ACF), to malignant tumors [2]. ACF are early focal lesions of the colonic mucosa composed of one to several enlarged crypts, which are specifically induced by colon carcinogens [3]. Easily identified in methylene blue-stained whole-mount preparations under a dissecting microscope, ACF are used as early indicators of colon carcinogenesis [1–3].
Cannabinoids have been licensed for clinical use as palliative treatment of chemotherapy, but increasing evidence shows antitumor actions of cannabinoid agonists on several tumor cells in vitro and in animal models."

Complete Study Link:
http://link.springer.com/article/10.1007%2Fs00109-007-0248-4

2008

Delta 9-tetrahydrocannabinol inhibits cell cycle progression by downregulation of E2F1 in human glioblastoma multiforme cells.

Acta Oncologica.

Galanti G, Fisher T, Kventsel I, Shoham J, Gallily R, Mechoulam R, Lavie G, Amariglio N, Rechavi G, Toren A.
The Mina and Everard Goodman Faculty of Life Science, Bar-Ilan University, Ramat-Gan, Israel.

Abstract

BACKGROUND:

The active components of Cannabis sativa L., Cannabinoids, traditionally used in the field of cancer for alleviation of pain, nausea, wasting and improvement of well-being have received renewed interest in recent years due to their diverse pharmacologic activities such as cell growth inhibition, anti-inflammatory activity and induction of tumor regression. Here we used several experimental approaches, which identified delta-9-tetrahydrocannabinol (Delta(9)-THC) as an essential mediator of cannabinoid antitumoral action.

METHODS AND RESULTS:

Administration of Delta(9)-THC to glioblastoma multiforme (GBM) cell lines results in a significant decrease in cell viability. Cell cycle analysis showed G(0/1) arrest and did not reveal occurrence of apoptosis in the absence of any sub-G(1) populations. Western blot analyses revealed a THC altered cellular content of proteins that regulate cell progression through the cell cycle. The cell content of E2F1 and Cyclin A, two proteins that promote cell cycle progression, were suppressed in both U251-MG and U87-MG human glioblastoma cell lines, whereas the level of p16(INK4A), a cell cycle inhibitor was upregulated. Transcription of thymidylate synthase (TS) mRNA, which is promoted by E2F1, also declined as evident by QRT-PCR. The decrease in E2F1 levels resulted from proteasome mediated degradation and was prevented by proteasome inhibitors.

CONCLUSIONS:

Delta(9)-THC is shown to significantly affect viability of GBM cells via a mechanism that appears to elicit G(1) arrest due to downregulation of E2F1 and Cyclin A. Hence, it is suggested that Delta(9)-THC and other cannabinoids be implemented in future clinical evaluation as a therapeutic modality for brain tumors.

PubMed Link: https://www.ncbi.nlm.nih.gov/pubmed/17934890

Expression and function of the endocannabinoid system in glial cells.

Current Pharmulactical Design.

Massi P, Valenti M, Bolognini D, Parolaro D.
Department of Structural and Functional Biology, Center of Neuroscience, University of Insubria, Busto Arsizio (VA), Italy.

Abstract

In the last few years the role and significance of the glia in CNS function and pathology have been drastically reassessed. Glial cells physiology appears very different in healthy versus pathological brain and the recent identification of cannabinoid receptors and their endogenous ligands in glia has triggered a number of studies exploring the role of (endo)cannabinoid system in glia functionality and disease. (Endo)cannabinoids exert their effects in these cells directly affecting some important peculiar functions of the glia and actively promoting biochemical signals ending in a pro-survival fate for these cells. By contrast, (endo)cannabinoids induce a selective death in glia-derived tumor cells. Of special physiological and therapeutic relevance is the reported ability of glial cells during neuropathological conditions to release an increased amount of endocannabinoids and to overexpress cannabinoid receptors. This evidence has suggested that the endocannabinoids production by glial cells may constitute an endogenous defense mechanism preventing the propagation of neuroinflammation and cell damage. The present paper will review the evidence supporting the regulatory role of (endo)cannabinoids in glia function, holding in consideration their therapeutic potential as neuroprotective and/or anticancer agents.

PubMed Link: https://www.ncbi.nlm.nih.gov/pubmed/18781979

Loss of cannabinoid receptor 1 accelerates intestinal tumor growth

Cancer Research.

Dingzhi Wang[1], Haibin Wang[2], Wei Ning[1], Michael G. Backlund[1], Sudhansu K. Dey[2,3,4], and Raymond N. DuBois[5,6]

[1] Department of Medicine, Vanderbilt University Medical Center, Nashville, TN

[2] Department of Pediatrics, Vanderbilt University Medical Center, Nashville, TN

[3] Department of Cancer Biology, Vanderbilt University Medical Center, Nashville, TN

[4] Department of Cell & Developmental Biology, Vanderbilt University Medical Center, Nashville, TN

[5] Vanderbilt-Ingram Cancer Center, Nashville, TN

[6] Departments of Gastrointestinal Oncology and Cancer Biology, The University of Texas MD Anderson Cancer Center, Houston, TX

Abstract

Although endocannabinoid signaling is important for certain aspects of gastrointestinal homoeostasis, the role of the cannabinoid receptors (CB) in colorectal cancer has not been defined. Here we show that CB1 expression was silenced in human colorectal cancer due to methylation of the CB1 promoter. Our genetic and pharmacologic studies reveal that loss or inhibition of CB1 accelerated intestinal adenoma growth in ApcMin/+ mice whereas activation of CB1 attenuatedintestinal tumor growth by inducing cell death via downregulation of the anti-apoptotic factor survivin. This downregulation of survivin by CB1 is mediated by a cAMP-dependent PKA signaling pathway. These results indicate that the endogenous cannabinoid system may represent a potential therapeutic target for prevention or treatment of colorectal cancer.

PubMed Links:

https://www.ncbi.nlm.nih.gov/pmc/articles/PMC2561258/
https://www.ncbi.nlm.nih.gov/pmc/articles/PMC2561258/pdf/nihms55091.pdf

Turned-off Cannabinoid Receptor Turns On Colorectal Tumor Growth

University of Texas M. D. Anderson Cancer Center

Summary: New preclinical research shows that cannabinoid cell surface receptor CB1 plays a tumor-suppressing role in human colorectal cancer, scientists report in the Aug. 1 edition of the Journal Cancer Research.

Link: https://www.sciencedaily.com/releases/2008/08/080801074056.htm

Cannabinoid receptor activation induces apoptosis through tumor necrosis factor alpha-mediated ceramide de novo synthesis in colon cancer cells.
Clinical Cancer Research.

Cianchi F, Papucci L, Schiavone N, Lulli M, Magnelli L, Vinci MC, Messerini L, Manera C, Ronconi E, Romagnani P, Donnini M, Perigli G, Trallori G, Tanganelli E, Capaccioli S, Masini E.
Department of Medical and Surgical Critical Care, University of Florence, Florence, Italy.

Abstract

PURPOSE:
Cannabinoids have been recently proposed as a new family of potential antitumor agents. The present study was undertaken to investigate the expression of the two cannabinoid receptors, CB1 and CB2, in colorectal cancer and to provide new insight into the molecular pathways underlying the apoptotic activity induced by their activation.
EXPERIMENTAL DESIGN:
Cannabinoid receptor expression was investigated in both human cancer specimens and in the DLD-1 and HT29 colon cancer cell lines. The effects of the CB1 agonist arachinodyl-2'-chloroethylamide and the CB2 agonist N-cyclopentyl-7-methyl-1-(2-morpholin-4-ylethyl)-1,8-naphthyridin-4(1H)-on-3-carboxamide (CB13) on tumor cell apoptosis and ceramide and tumor necrosis factor (TNF)-alpha production were evaluated. The knock-down of TNF-alpha mRNA was obtained with the use of selective small interfering RNA.
RESULTS:
We show that the CB1 receptor was mainly expressed in human normal colonic epithelium whereas tumor tissue was strongly positive for the CB2 receptor. The activation of the CB1 and, more efficiently, of the CB2 receptors induced apoptosis and increased ceramide levels in the DLD-1 and HT29 cells. Apoptosis was prevented by the pharmacologic inhibition of ceramide de novo synthesis. The CB2 agonist CB13 also reduced the growth of DLD-1 cells in a mouse model of colon cancer. The knockdown of TNF-alpha mRNA abrogated the ceramide increase and, therefore, the apoptotic effect induced by cannabinoid receptor activation.
CONCLUSIONS:
The present study shows that either CB1 or CB2 receptor activation induces apoptosis through ceramide de novo synthesis in colon cancer cells. Our data unveiled, for the first time, that TNF-alpha acts as a link between cannabinoid receptor activation and ceramide production.

PubMed Link: https://www.ncbi.nlm.nih.gov/pubmed/19047095

FROM FULL TEXT:

"There is growing evidence that cannabinoids may selectively target tumor cells by the activation of their membrane receptors, CB1 and CB2. However, the mechanisms underlying the antitumor effects of this activation are still not well understood, and experimental data suggest that these effects may be cell-type

124

specific. The regulation of the RAS–mitogenactivated protein kinase/extracellular signal-regulated kinase (MAPK/ERK) and the phosphatidylinositol 3-kinase–AKT pathways and the stimulation of ceramide synthesis are among the mechanisms proposed to explain the antitumor effects of cannabinoids in different types of human cancer (reviewed in refs. 5, 6). Indeed, these pathways have been reported to be differently triggered depending on the tumor cell type investigated. In the present study, we report that both CB1 and CB2 cannabinoid receptor activation induces apoptosis in colon cancer cells, and this is mediated by the de novo synthesis of ceramide."

Complete Study Links:

http://clincancerres.aacrjournals.org/content/14/23/7691.long
http://clincancerres.aacrjournals.org/content/clincanres/14/23/7691.full.pdf

A high cannabinoid CB(1) receptor immunoreactivity is associated with disease severity and outcome in prostate cancer.

European Journal of Cancer.

Sui Chu Chunga, Peter Hammarstenb, Andreas Josefssonb, Pä r Stattinc, Torvald Granforsd,
Lars Egevade, Giacomo Mancinif, Beat Lutzf, Anders Berghb,
Christopher J. Fowlera,

aDepartment of Pharmacology and Clinical Neuroscience, Pharmacology, Umea° University, Umea° , Sweden
bDepartment of Medical Biosciences, Pathology, Umea° University, Umea° , Sweden
cDepartment of Surgical and Perioperative Sciences, Urology and Andrology, Umea° University, Umea° , Sweden
dDepartment of Urology, Central Hospital, Va¨ stera° s, Sweden
eInternational Agency for Research on Cancer, Lyon, France
fDepartment of Physiological Chemistry, Johannes Gutenberg-University Mainz, Mainz, Germany

Abstract

In the light of findings indicating that cannabinoids can affect the proliferation of a number of cancer cell types and that cannabinoid receptor expression is higher in prostate cancer cell lines than in non-malignant cells, we investigated whether the level of cannabinoid 1 receptor immunoreactivity (CB(1)IR) in prostate cancer tissues is associated with disease severity and outcome. Formalin-fixed paraffin-embedded non-malignant and tumour tissue samples from patients who were diagnosed with prostate cancer at a transurethral resection for voiding problems were used. CB(1)IR, which was scored in a total of 399 cases, was associated with the epithelial cell membranes, with little staining in the stroma. Patients with a tumour CB(1)IR score greater or equal to the median (2) had a significantly higher proportion of Gleason scores 8-10, metastases at diagnosis, tumour size and rate of cell proliferation at diagnosis than patients with a score<2. For 269 cases, tumour CB(1)IR was measured for patients who only received palliative therapy at the end stages of the disease,

125

allowing the influence of CB(1)IR upon the disease outcome to be determined. Receiver operating characteristic (ROC) curves showed an area under the curve of 0.67 (95% confidence limits 0.59-0.74) for CB(1)IR in the tumour. CB(1)IR in non-malignant tissue was not associated with disease outcome. A tumour CB(1)IR score >or=2 was associated with a significantly lower disease specific survival. A Cox proportional hazards regression indicated that the tumour CB(1)IR score and the Gleason score were independent prognostic variables. It is concluded that a high tumour CB(1)IR score is associated with prostate cancer severity and outcome.

PubMed Link: https://www.ncbi.nlm.nih.gov/pubmed/19056257

FROM FULL TEXT:

"Prostate cancer is the major cancer form afflicting males. In the United States of America (USA), for example, the American Cancer Society listed 218,219 new cancer cases in their estimates for 2007, a number approximately equal to the number of male cases for lung and bronchus, colon and rectum, and melanoma of the skin put together.1 There is a wide range of treatment options for prostate cancer depending on tumour characteristics, patient age and status. However, the curative treatments for localised prostate cancer (prostatectomy and radiation therapy) are associated with the risks of side-effects, including erectile dysfunction and incontinence,2–4 and both novel treatment strategies and prognostic markers (to avoid the overtreatment of patients who would better have been served by surveillance alone5) are much needed. D9-Tetrahydrocannabinol (D9-THC), the main psychoactive ingredient of cannabis, produces most of its effects via the activation of two G-protein coupled cannabinoid (CB) receptors termed CB1 and CB2. CB1 receptors are among the most common of all receptor types in the brain, and are also located peripherally in both neurons and non-neuronal tissue, whilst CB2 receptors are mainly found in immune cells.6 The endogenous ligands for these receptors ('endocannabinoids') anandamide and 2-arachidonoylglycerol are synthesised on demand and mimic many of the actions of D9-THC, but have short-lived effects due to effective metabolic pathways.7,8 Synthetic D9-THC (MarinolTM) and its analogue nabilone (CesametTM) are licensed in the USA, Canada and the United Kingdom (UK) for their palliative effects upon chemotherapy- induced nausea and vomiting. However, cannabinoids also affect the viability, proliferation, adhesion and migration of cancer cells, including prostate cancer cells, and can reduce angiogenesis and the growth of tumour cells implanted into nude mice."

Complete Study Links:
http://www.ejcancer.com/article/S0959-8049%2808%2900810-1/fulltext
http://www.ejcancer.com/article/S0959-8049%2808%2900810-1/pdf

Cannabinoid 2 receptor induction by IL-12 and its potential as a therapeutic target for the treatment of anaplastic thyroid carcinoma.

Cancer Gene Therapy.

Shi Y, Zou M, Baitei EY, Alzahrani AS, Parhar RS, Al-Makhalafi Z, Al-Mohanna FA.

Department of Genetics, King Faisal Specialist Hospital and Research Center, Riyadh, Saudi Arabia.

Abstract

Anaplastic thyroid carcinoma is the most aggressive type of thyroid malignancies. Previously, we demonstrated that tumorigenicity of anaplastic thyroid carcinoma cell line ARO was significantly reduced following interleukin (IL)-12 gene transfer. We suspected that tumor target structure in ARO/IL-12 cells might be changed and such a change may make them more susceptible to be killed through mechanisms apart from natural killer-dependent pathway. To identify genes involved, we examined gene expression profile of ARO and ARO/IL-12 by microarray analysis of 3757 genes. The most highly expressed gene was cannabinoid receptor 2 (CB2), which was expressed eightfold higher in ARO/IL-12 cells than ARO cells. CB2 agonist JWH133 and mixed CB1/CB2 agonist WIN-55,212-2 could induce significantly higher rate of apoptosis in ARO/IL-12 than ARO cells. Similar results were obtained when ARO cells were transfected with CB2 transgene (ARO/CB2). A considerable regression of thyroid tumors generated by inoculation of ARO/CB2 cells was observed in nude mice following local administration of JWH133. We also demonstrated significant increase in the induction of apoptosis in ARO/IL12 and ARO/CB2 cells following incubation with 15 nM paclitaxel, indicating that tumor cells were sensitized to chemotherapy. These data suggest that CB2 overexpression may contribute to the regression of human anaplastic thyroid tumor in nude mice following IL-12 gene transfer. Given that cannabinoids have shown antitumor effects in many types of cancer models, CB2 may be a viable therapeutic target for the treatment of anaplastic thyroid carcinoma.

PubMed Link: https://www.ncbi.nlm.nih.gov/pubmed/18197164

FROM FULL TEXT:

"Numerous reports have indicated that cannabinoids, the active components of Cannabis sativa (marijuana) and their derivatives, can inhibit cancer cell growth, angiogenesis, invasion and metastasis by modulating key cell-signalling pathways, such as MAPKs and phosphatidylinositol 3-kinase pathways,17, 18, 19, 20 both of which have been involved in thyroid carcinoma.21 For example, multiple genetic defects were found in the RET/PTC(TRK)–RAS–BRAF–MEK–MAPK kinase pathway. The most frequent one was BRAF mutation: 44% found in papillary thyroid carcinoma and 24% in anaplastic thyroid carcinoma.22 BRAF mutation would lead to increased phosphorylated pERK protein expression. Recent study has shown that Δ9-tetrahydrocannabinol, the major psychoactive ingredient of marijuana, can downregulate genes involved in this pathway, resulting in decreased phosphorylated pERK protein expression.23 Although the evidence for its medical use is compelling, its legal or licensed use in medicine is still a controversial issue in most countries due to widespread illegal use of cannabis as a recreational drug."

Complete Study Links:
http://www.nature.com/cgt/journal/v15/n2/full/7701101a.html
http://www.nature.com/cgt/journal/v15/n2/pdf/7701101a.pdf

Estrogenic induction of cannabinoid CB1 receptor in human colon cancer cell lines.

Scandinavian Journal of Gastroenterology.
Notarnicola M, Messa C, Orlando A, Bifulco M,
Laezza C, Gazzerro P, Caruso MG.
Laboratory of Biochemistry, National Institute for Digestive Diseases S. de Bellis, Castellana Grotte, Bari, Italy.

Abstract

OBJECTIVE:

Cannabinoids are a class of compounds that have the ability to activate two specific receptor subtypes, the cannabinoid CB1 and CB2 receptors. CB1 receptor is a G-protein-coupled receptor that is linked to the signal transduction pathways. The cumulative effects of this receptor have important implications in the control of cell survival and cell death having the potential to regulate tumor cell growth. In this connection, interest has been focused on factors such as sex steroid hormones, which regulate CB1 receptor expression. The aim of this study was to investigate the effects of 17beta-estradiol exposure on the CB1 receptor gene and its protein expression in human primary tumor colon cancer cell lines, such as DLD-1, HT-29 and one lymph node metastatic cell line, SW620.

MATERIAL AND METHODS:

CB1 gene expression was determined using quantitative reverse transcriptase-polymerase chain reaction (RT-PCR) in DLD-1, HT-29 and SW620 cells treated at different times and doses of 17beta-estradiol exposure. CB 1 protein expression was detected by Western immunoblot.

RESULTS:

17beta-estradiol induced CB1 gene expression in all the human colon cancer cells studied. The early induction of CB1 receptor mRNA in DLD-1 and SW620 cells was mediated by the estrogen receptor because the pure estrogen antagonist, ICI 182,780, was able to counteract this effect. Estrogenic induction of the CB1 receptor was also detectable at protein level in all cell types tested.

CONCLUSIONS:

The CB1 receptor can be considered an estrogen-responsive gene in DLD-1, HT-29 and SW620 cells. Up-regulation of CB1 expression by 17beta-estradiol is a further mechanism of estrogens to control colon cancer proliferation.

PubMed Link: https://www.ncbi.nlm.nih.gov/pubmed/18938775

"Plant-derived, synthetic or endogenous cannabinoids are a class of compounds that have the ability to activate two specific receptors subtypes, the cannabinoid CB1 and CB2 receptors. CB1 receptors, first detected in brain, have also been detected in reproductive tissues and the gastrointestinal system [1,2], whereas CB2 receptors appear to be expressed mainly by cells of the immune system [2]. The CB1 receptor is a G-protein-coupled receptor that is linked to signal transduction pathways including inhibition of adenylate cyclase, activation of mitogen-activated protein kinase and regulation of calcium and potassium channels [2]. The cumulative effects of this receptor have important implications in the control of cell survival and cell death having the potential to regulate tumor cell growth....

The present findings suggest that the anti-proliferative action of 17b-estradiol on human colon cancer cells may also be related to its ability to induce CB1 receptor expression. Estrogenic regulation of the CB1 receptor gene in colon cancer cell lines, detected in this study, concurs with the results of recent studies showing that both CB1 receptor gene expression and the FAAH enzyme are influenced by estrogen in the human anterior pituitary gland and in mouse endometrial epithelium, respectively [11,22]....

Up-regulation of the endocannabinoid system by estrogens is a further mechanism of growth control in colon cancer; therefore, the use of estrogens in an anti-cancer therapeutic strategy has to be encouraged. Finally, the activation of synthesis of endocannabinoids and their receptors, as well as the inactivation of their enzymatic hydrolysis might be important in a strategy for developing new anticancer drugs."

Complete Study   Link:

https://www.researchgate.net/publication/23400468_Estrogenic_induction_of_cannabinoid_CB1_receptor_in_human_colon_cancer_cell_lines

Cannabinoids for cancer treatment: progress and promise.

Cancer Research.

Sarfaraz S, Adhami VM, Syed DN, Afaq F, Mukhtar H.
Chemoprevention Program, Paul P. Carbone Comprehensive Cancer Center and Department of Dermatology, School of Medicine and Public Health, University of Wisconsin, Madison, Wisconsin, USA.

Abstract
Cannabinoids are a class of pharmacologic compounds that offer potential applications as antitumor drugs, based on the ability of some members of this class to limit inflammation, cell proliferation, and cell survival. In particular, emerging evidence suggests that agonists of cannabinoid receptors expressed by tumor cells may offer a novel strategy to treat cancer. Here, we review recent work that raises interest in the development and exploration of potent, nontoxic, and nonhabit forming cannabinoids for cancer therapy.

PubMed Link: https://www.ncbi.nlm.nih.gov/pubmed/18199524

"Although there are few contradictory studies on the mechanism of action of cannabinoids, they all underline the importance of cannabinoids for the treatment of cancer. Hence, further studies are needed to elucidate the mechanism of action of cannabinoids in cancer treatment. Cannabinoids, the active components of marijuana and their other natural and synthetic analogues have been reported as useful adjuvants to conventional chemotherapeutic regimens for preventing nausea, vomiting, pain, and for stimulating appetite. Before the discovery of specific cannabinoid systems and receptors, it was speculated that cannabinoids produced their effects via nonspecific interaction with cell membranes. Cannabinoids are proving to be unique based on their targeted action on cancer cells and their ability to spare normal cells. Variation in the effects of cannabinoids in different cell lines and tumor model could be due to the differential expression of CB1 and CB2 receptors. Thus, overexpression of cannabinoid receptors may be effective in killing tumors, whereas low or no expression of these receptors could lead to cell proliferation and metastasis because of the suppression of the antitumor immune response. It is also reported that low doses of cannabinoid administration accelerate proliferation of cancer cells instead of inducing apoptosis and, thereby, contribute to cancer progression. Till date, very little is known about the mechanism of action of cannabinoids. There is need for further in-depth studies to elucidate the precise mechanism of cannabinoid action in cancer cells. Safety of D(9)-tetrahydrocannabinol administration has been determined, and a dose escalation regimen showed that cannabinoid delivery was safe and could be achieved without overt psychoactive effects. In view of the fair safety profile of most cannabinoids together with their antiproliferative action on tumor cells, clinical trials are required to determine whether cannabinoids could be used for the inhibition of tumor growth in a clinical setting."

Complete Study Links:

http://cancerres.aacrjournals.org/content/68/2/339.long
http://cancerres.aacrjournals.org/content/canres/68/2/339.full.pdf

Inhibition of cancer cell invasion by cannabinoids via increased expression of tissue inhibitor of matrix metalloproteinases-1.

Journal National Cancer Inst.
Ramer R, Hinz B.
Institute of Toxicology and Pharmacology, University of Rostock, Schillingallee 70, Rostock, Germany.

Abstract
BACKGROUND:
Cannabinoids, in addition to having palliative benefits in cancer therapy, have been associated with anticarcinogenic effects. Although the antiproliferative activities of can-

nabinoids have been intensively investigated, little is known about their effects on tumor invasion.

METHODS:

Matrigel-coated and uncoated Boyden chambers were used to quantify invasiveness and migration, respectively, of human cervical cancer (HeLa) cells that had been treated with cannabinoids (the stable anandamide analog R(+)-methanandamide [MA] and the phyto-cannabinoid delta9-tetrahydrocannabinol [THC]) in the presence or absence of antagonists of the CB1 or CB2 cannabinoid receptors or of transient receptor potential vanilloid 1 (TRPV1) or inhibitors of p38 or p42/44 mitogen-activated protein kinase (MAPK) pathways. Reverse transcriptase-polymerase chain reaction (RT-PCR) and immunoblotting were used to assess the influence of cannabinoids on the expression of matrix metalloproteinases (MMPs) and endogenous tissue inhibitors of MMPs (TIMPs). The role of TIMP-1 in the anti-invasive action of cannabinoids was analyzed by transfecting HeLa, human cervical carcinoma (C33A), or human lung carcinoma cells (A549) cells with siRNA targeting TIMP-1. All statistical tests were two-sided.

RESULTS:

Without modifying migration, MA and THC caused a time- and concentration-dependent suppression of HeLa cell invasion through Matrigel that was accompanied by increased expression of TIMP-1. At the lowest concentrations tested, MA (0.1 microM) and THC (0.01 microM) led to a decrease in invasion (normalized to that observed with vehicle-treated cells) of 61.5% (95% CI = 38.7% to 84.3%, P < .001) and 68.1% (95% CI = 31.5% to 104.8%, P = .0039), respectively. The stimulation of TIMP-1 expression and suppression of cell invasion were reversed by pretreatment of cells with antagonists to CB1 or CB2 receptors, with inhibitors of MAPKs, or, in the case of MA, with an antagonist to TRPV1. Knockdown of cannabinoid-induced TIMP-1 expression by siRNA led to a reversal of the cannabinoid-elicited decrease in tumor cell invasiveness in HeLa, A549, and C33A cells.

CONCLUSION:

Increased expression of TIMP-1 mediates an anti-invasive effect of cannabinoids. Cannabinoids may therefore offer a therapeutic option in the treatment of highly invasive cancers.

PubMed Link: https://www.ncbi.nlm.nih.gov/pubmed/18159069

FROM FULL TEXT:

"There is considerable evidence to suggest an important role for cannabinoids in conferring anticarcinogenic activities. In this study, we identified TIMP-1 as a mediator of the anti-invasive actions of MA, a hydrolysis-stable analog of the endocannabinoid anandamide, and THC, a plant-derived cannabinoid. Both cannabinoids decreased HeLa cell invasion in a time- and concentration-dependent manner. Following a 72-hour incubation, the decrease of invasiveness by MA and THC was statistically significant at concentrations as low as 0.1 μ M and 0.01 μ M (at these concentrations we observed 61.5% inhibition of invasion by MA and 68.1% inhibition by THC). In humans, average peak plasma concentrations of THC of 0.03 μ M and 0.045 μ M could be achieved with oral doses of 15 and 20 mg, respectively (38) and were associated with a statistically significant reduction of cancer pain (39,40). Thus, effects of THC on cell invasion occurred at therapeutically relevant concentrations.

Our finding that reduced invasion was not associated with decreased cellular motility suggested that the reduction in invasiveness that was observed when cells were treated with cannabinoids was a specific effect that was dependent on the modulation of matrix-degrading enzymes. Although this result rules out a decisive role of migration in mediating the anti-invasive action of cannabinoids in our system, others have reported antimigrative properties of cannabinoids that suggest that these substances affect migration in a cell type – specific and/or chemoattractant- dependent manner. For example, in human breast cancer cells, cannabinoid treatment inhibits adhesion and migration on type IV collagen,

possibly via decreased tyrosine phosphorylation of focal adhesion kinase (44). Furthermore, a cannabinoid receptor – independent mechanism was proposed to underlie the antimigrative action of cannabidiol on human glioma cells (45)....

In conclusion, our results suggest that there exists a signaling pathway by which the binding of cannabinoids to specifi c receptors leads via intracellular MAPK activation to induction of TIMP-1 expression and subsequent inhibition of tumor cell invasion. To our knowledge, this is the first report of TIMP-1 – dependent antiinvasive effects of cannabinoids. This signaling pathway may play an important role in the antimetastatic action of cannabinoids, whose potential therapeutic benefit in the treatment of highly invasive cancers should be addressed in clinical trials."

Complete Study Links:
http://jnci.oxfordjournals.org/content/100/1/59.long
http://jnci.oxfordjournals.org/content/100/1/59.full.pdf

Cannabinoid receptor-independent cytotoxic effects of cannabinoids in human colorectal carcinoma cells: synergism with 5-fluorouracil.

Cancer Chemotherapy Pharmacology.

Gustafsson SB, Lindgren T, Jonsson M, Jacobsson SO.
Department of Pharmacology and Clinical Neuroscience, Umeå University, Umea, Sweden.

Abstract

Cannabinoids (CBs) have been found to exert antiproliferative effects upon a variety of cancer cells, including colorectal carcinoma cells. However, little is known about the signalling mechanisms behind the antitumoural effect in these cells, whether the effects are shared by endogenous lipids related to endocannabinoids, or whether such effects are synergistic with treatment paradigms currently used in the clinic. The aim of this preclinical study was to investigate the effect of synthetic and endogenous CBs and their related fatty acids on the viability of human colorectal carcinoma Caco-2 cells, and to determine whether CB effects are synergistic with those seen with the pyrimidine antagonist 5-fluorouracil (5-FU). The synthetic CB HU 210, the endogenous CB anandamide, the endogenous structural analogue of anandamide, N-arachidonoyl glycine (NAGly), as well as the related polyunsaturated fatty acids arachidonic acid and eicosapentaenoic acid showed antiproliferative and cytotoxic effects in the Caco-2 cells, as measured by using

[(3)H]-thymidine incorporation assay, the CyQUANT proliferation assay and calcein-AM fluorescence. HU 210 was the most potent compound examined, followed by anandamide, whereas NAGly showed equal potency and efficacy as the polyunsaturated fatty acids. Furthermore, HU 210 and 5-FU produced synergistic effects in the Caco-2 cells, but not in the human colorectal carcinoma cell lines HCT116 or HT29. The compounds examined produced cytotoxic, rather than antiproliferative effects, by a mechanism not involving CB receptors, since the CB receptor antagonists AM251 and AM630 did not attenuate the effects, nor did pertussis toxin. However, alpha-tocopherol and the nitric oxide synthase inhibitor L-NAME attenuated the CB toxicity, suggesting involvement of oxidative stress. It is concluded that the CB system may provide new targets for the development of drugs to treat colorectal cancer.

PubMed Link: https://www.ncbi.nlm.nih.gov/pubmed/18629502

Endocannabinoids in endocrine and related tumours.
Endocrine Relatated Cancer.

Bifulco M, Malfitano AM, Pisanti S, Laezza C.
Dipartimento di Scienze Farmaceutiche, Università di Salerno, Fisciano (Salerno), Italy IEOS, CNR Napoli, Italy.

Abstract
The 'endocannabinoid system', comprising the cannabinoid CB1 and CB2 receptors, their endogenous ligands, endocannabinoids and the enzymes that regulate their biosynthesis and degradation, has drawn a great deal of scientist attention during the last two decades. The endocannabinoid system is involved in a broad range of functions and in a growing number of physiopathological conditions. Indeed, recent evidence indicates that endocannabinoids influence the intracellular events controlling the proliferation of numerous types of endocrine and related cancer cells, thereby leading to both in vitro and in vivo antitumour effects. In particular, they are able to inhibit cell growth, invasion and metastasis of thyroid, breast and prostate tumours. The chief events of endocannabinoids in cancer cell proliferation are reported highlighting the correspondent signalling involved in tumour processes: regulation of adenylyl cyclase, cyclic AMP-protein kinase-A pathway and MEK-extracellular signal-regulated kinase signalling cascade.

PubMed Link: https://www.ncbi.nlm.nih.gov/pubmed/18508995

FROM FULL TEXT:

"Accumulated evidence indicates that CBs could be an important target for the treatment of cancer due to their ability to regulate signalling pathways critical for cell growth and survival. Several studies have produced exciting new leads in the search for anticancer treatments with cannabinoid-related drugs. Natural, THC, synthetic, HU210, WIN-55,212-2 and endogenous, 2-AG, AEA cannabinoids are nowadays known to control various cancer types by modulating tumour growth, apoptosis, migration and blood supply to tumours (Bifulco & Di Marzo 2002, Guzman et al. 2002)."

Complete Study Links:
http://erc.endocrinology-journals.org/content/15/2/391.long
http://erc.endocrinology-journals.org/content/15/2/391.full.pdf

Expression of cannabinoid receptors type 1 and type 2 in non-Hodgkin lymphoma: growth inhibition by receptor activation.

International Journal of Cancer.

Gustafsson K, Wang X, Severa D, Eriksson M, Kimby E, Merup M, Christensson B, Flygare J, Sander B.

Department of Laboratory Medicine, Division of Pathology, Karolinska Institutet and Karolinska University Hospital Huddinge, Stockholm, Sweden.

Abstract

Endogenous and synthetic cannabinoids exert antiproliferative and proapoptotic effects in various types of cancer and in mantle cell lymphoma (MCL). In this study, we evaluated the expression of cannabinoid receptors type 1 and type 2 (CB1 and CB2) in non-Hodgkin lymphomas of B cell type (n = 62). A majority of the lymphomas expressed higher mRNA levels of CB1 and/or CB2 as compared to reactive lymphoid tissue. With the exception of MCL, which uniformly overexpresses both CB1 and CB2, the levels of cannabinoid receptors within other lymphoma entities were highly variable, ranging from 0.1 to 224 times the expression in reactive lymph nodes. Low levels of the splice variant CB1a, previously shown to have a different affinity for cannabinoids than CB1, were detected in 44% of the lymphomas, while CB1b expression was not detected. In functional studies using MCL, Burkitt lymphoma (BL), chronic lymphatic leukemia (CLL) and plasma cell leukemia cell lines, the stable anandamide analog R(+)-methanandamide (R(+)-MA) induced cell death only in MCL and CLL cells, which overexpressed both cannabinoid receptors, but not in BL. In vivo treatment with R(+)-MA caused a significant reduction of tumor size and mitotic index in mice xenografted with human MCL. Together, our results suggest that therapies using cannabinoid receptor ligands will have efficiency in reducing tumor burden in malignant lymphoma overexpressing CB1 and CB2.

PubMed Link: https://www.ncbi.nlm.nih.gov/pubmed/18546271

FROM FULL TEXT:

"Our results show that CB1 and CB2 are expressed in several entities of non Hodgkin lymphomas of B cell type. The highly variable expression within well-defined lymphoma entities suggests that cannabinoid receptors may be potential targets for individualized therapeutic interventions. Treatment with the stable endocannabinoid analog R(+)-MA induces apoptosis in tumor cell lines from MCL and CLL, expressing higher levels of both CB1 and CB2 compared with reactive lymphoid tissue. Furthermore, decreased growth of MCL in vivo was observed following intratumoral injections of R(+)-MA. Similarly, in studies using animal models or xenografts of breast, lung cancer, skin, prostate and brain cancer, anti-tumor effects by cannabinoids have been reported (reviewed in Refs. 19 and 20). In a pilot study on patients with glioblastoma multiforme, Δ9-tetrahydrocannabinol reduced tumor cell proliferation in vivo.34 These cumulative data suggest that targeting of the endocannabinoid system could possibly be part of a future therapy for certain malignant lymphomas as has been suggested for other forms of cancer."

Complete Study Links:

http://onlinelibrary.wiley.com/doi/10.1002/ijc.23584/full
http://onlinelibrary.wiley.com/doi/10.1002/ijc.23584/pdf

Cannabinoids inhibit glioma cell invasion by down-regulating matrix metalloproteinase-2 expression.
Cancer Research.

Blázquez C, Salazar M, Carracedo A, Lorente M, Egia A, González-Feria L, Haro A, Velasco G, Guzmán M.
Department of Biochemistry and Molecular Biology I, School of Biology, Complutense University, Madrid, Spain.

Abstract

Cannabinoids, the active components of Cannabis sativa L. and their derivatives, inhibit tumor growth in laboratory animals by inducing apoptosis of tumor cells and impairing tumor angiogenesis. It has also been reported that these compounds inhibit tumor cell spreading, but the molecular targets of this cannabinoid action remain elusive. Here, we evaluated the effect of cannabinoids on matrix metalloproteinase (MMP) expression and its effect on tumor cell invasion. Local administration of Delta(9)-tetrahydrocannabinol (THC), the major active ingredient of cannabis, down-regulated MMP-2 expression in gliomas generated in mice, as determined by Western blot, immunofluorescence, and real-time quantitative PCR analyses. This cannabinoid-induced inhibition of MMP-2 expression in gliomas (a) was MMP-2-selective, as levels of other MMP family members were unaffected; (b) was mimicked by JWH-133, a CB(2) cannabinoid receptor-selective agonist that is devoid of psychoactive side effects; (c) was abrogated by fumonisin B1, a selective inhibitor of ceramide biosynthesis; and (d) was also evident in two patients with recurrent glioblastoma multiforme. THC inhibited MMP-2 expression and cell invasion in cultured glioma cells. Manipulation of MMP-2 expression by RNA interference and cDNA overexpression experiments proved that down-regulation of this MMP plays a critical role in THC-mediated inhibition of cell invasion. Cannabinoid-induced inhibition of MMP-2 expression and cell invasion was prevented by blocking ceramide biosynthesis and by knocking-down the expression of the stress protein p8. As MMP-2 up-regulation is associated with high progression and poor prognosis of gliomas and many other tumors, MMP-2 down-regulation constitutes a new hallmark of cannabinoid antitumoral activity.

PubMed Link: https://www.ncbi.nlm.nih.gov/pubmed/18339876

FROM FULL TEXT:

"THC inhibits MMP-2 expression in mouse gliomas. To test whether cannabinoid administration affects MMP levels, we generated subcutaneous gliomas in mice. The specificity of cannabinoid action was ascertained by the parallel study of C6.9 and C6.4 glioma cells, which constitute well-established models of cannabinoid-responsive and cannabinoid-resistant cells, respectively (7, 10, 23). Tumors were treated with either vehicle or THC and MMP levels were determined by Western blot. Cannabinoid administration decreased tumor growth (Fig. 1A) and MMP-2 expression (Fig. 1B) in C6.9-cell gliomas."

Complete Study Links:

http://cancerres.aacrjournals.org/content/68/6/1945
http://cancerres.aacrjournals.org/content/canres/68/6/1945.full.pdf

JunD is involved in the antiproliferative effect of Delta9-tetrahydrocannabinol on human breast cancer cells.

Oncogene.
Caffarel MM, Moreno-Bueno G, Cerutti C, Palacios J, Guzman M, Mechta-Grigoriou F, Sanchez C.
Department of Biochemistry and Molecular Biology I, School of Biology, Complutense University, Madrid, Spain.

Abstract

It has been recently shown that cannabinoids, the active components of marijuana and their derivatives, inhibit cell cycle progression of human breast cancer cells. Here we studied the mechanism of Delta(9)-tetrahydrocannabinol (THC) antiproliferative action in these cells, and show that it involves the modulation of JunD, a member of the AP-1 transcription factor family. THC activates JunD both by upregulating gene expression and by translocating the protein to the nuclear compartment, and these events are accompanied by a decrease in cell proliferation. Of interest, neither JunD activation nor proliferation inhibition was observed in human non-tumour mammary epithelial cells exposed to THC. We confirmed the importance of JunD in THC action by RNA interference and genetic ablation. Thus, in both JunD-silenced human breast cancer cells and JunD knockout mice-derived immortalized fibroblasts, the antiproliferative effect exerted by THC was significantly diminished. Gene array and siRNA experiments support that the cyclin-dependent kinase inhibitor p27 and the tumour suppressor gene testin are candidate JunD targets in cannabinoid action. In addition, our data suggest that the stress-regulated protein p8 participates in THC antiproliferative action in a JunD-independent manner. In summary, this is the first report showing not only that cannabinoids regulate JunD but, more generally, that JunD activation reduces the proliferation of cancer cells, which points to a new target to inhibit breast cancer progression.

PubMed Link: https://www.ncbi.nlm.nih.gov/pubmed/18454173

FROM FULL TEXT:

There is increasing evidence that cannabinoids, the active components of marijuana and their derivatives, possess antitumoural properties. Thus, a wide variety of cannabinoid compounds, including Δ9-tetrahydrocannabinol (THC, the most abundant and potent plant-derived cannabinoid) and other phytocannabinoids (cannabinol, cannabidiol), endocannabinoids (endogenously produced cannabinoids) and synthetic cannabinoids, exerts antiproliferative actions on a wide spectrum of tumour cells in vitro (Guzman, 2003). This effect has been confirmed in animal models of lung, pancreas, skin and breast carcinomas, glioma, thyroid epithelioma, lymphoma and melanoma (Guzman, 2003; Blazquez et al., 2006; Carracedo et al., 2006a; Ligresti et al., 2006). Cannabinoids exert most of their antiproliferative actions through activation of specific G-protein-coupled receptors. So far, two cannabinoid receptors—CB1 and CB2—have been cloned and characterized from mammalian tissues (Guzman, 2003). They differ mainly in their tissue-expression pattern: although CB1 is mostly present in the brain, peripheral nerve terminals and other non-neural sites such as testis, eye, vascular endothelium and spleen, CB2 expression is almost restricted to the immune system (Guzman, 2003). Engagement of these receptors modulates signalling pathways critically involved in the control of cell growth and survival (Guzman, 2003). It has been proposed that cannabinoids exert their antiproliferative effects on human breast cancer cells (HBCCs), at least in part, by controlling the progression through the cell cycle (De Petrocellis et al., 1998; Caffarel et al., 2006; Sarnataro et al., 2006). In particular, THC induces cell-cycle arrest at the G2–M transition by downregulating cyclin-dependent kinase 1 (CDK1, Cdc2) (Caffarel et al., 2006). However, the molecular bases of this cannabinoid effect are as yet unknown. Here we therefore investigated the mechanism underlying cannabinoid antiproliferative action in HBCCs.

Complete Study Links:

http://www.nature.com/onc/journal/v27/n37/full/onc2008145a.html
http://www.nature.com/onc/journal/v27/n37/pdf/onc2008145a.pdf

The endocannabinoid anandamide neither impairs in vitro T-cell function nor induces regulatory T-cell generation.

Anticancer Research.

Lissoni P, Tintori A, Fumagalli L, Brivio F, Messina G, Parolini D, Biondi A, Balestra A, D'Amico G.
Division of Radiation Oncology, Clinica Pediatrica Università Milano-Bicocca, Ospedale San Gerardo, Monza, Italy.

Abstract

BACKGROUND:

The cannabinoids have been proposed in the treatment of cancer. Generally, the cannabinoids are believed to be useful only in the palliative therapy of cancer-related symptoms, namely pain, anorexia and cachexia. However, preliminary experiments would also suggest an inhibitory effect of cannabinoids on cancer growth, whereas their influence on anticancer immunity is still controversial. The present study aimed to evaluate the influence of the endogenous cannabinoid anandamide (AEA) on T-cell phenotype and function.

MATERIALS AND METHODS:

The in vitro effects of AEA were evaluated at different concentrations on lymphocyte proliferation, cytotoxicity and differentiation, and in particular on T-regulator generation.

RESULTS:

AEA did not modify lymphocyte proliferation, neither under basal conditions, nor after IL-2 stimulation. Moreover, AEA did not induce the generation of regulatory T-lymphocytes nor the production of the immunosuppressive cytokine, IL-IO.

CONCLUSION:

The direct antitumor activity of AEA together with the absence of negative effects on T-cell functions might provide new insights into the potential use of cannabinoid agents in cancer immunotherapy.

PubMed Link: https://www.ncbi.nlm.nih.gov/pubmed/19189659

FROM FULL TEXT:

"The opioid substances have been proven to stimulate cancer cell proliferation (7, 8) and to inhibit the anticancer immune response (9). On the contrary, the cannabinoid molecules appear to inhibit the proliferation of several tumorbhistotypes (10, 11), to have antiangiogenic role (12) and to inhibit tumor cell migration (13). Several studies have demonstrated a significant antitumoral action of cannabinoid ligands in animal models (14). Thus, cannabinoid administration to nude mice curbs the growth of different tumors, including gliomas, lung adenocarcinomas, thyroid epitheliomas, lymphomas and skin carcinomas (14)."

Complete Study Links:

http://ar.iiarjournals.org/content/28/6A/3743.long
http://ar.iiarjournals.org/content/28/6A/3743.full.pdf

2009

. Changes in the endocannabinoid system may give insight into new and effective treatments for cancer.

Vitamins and Hormones

Alpini G, Demorrow S.
Department of Medicine, Texas A&M Health Science Center, College of Medicine, Temple, Texas, USA.

Abstract

The endocannabinoid system comprises specific cannabinoid receptors such as Cb1 and Cb2, the endogenous ligands (anandamide and 2-arachidonyl glycerol among others) and the proteins responsible for their synthesis and degradation. This system has become the focus of research in recent years because of its potential therapeutic value several disease states. The following review describes our current knowledge of the changes that occur in the endocannabinoid system during carcinogenesis and then focuses on the effects of anandamide on various aspects of the carcinogenic process such as growth, migration, and angiogenesis in tumors from various origins.

PubMed Link: https://www.ncbi.nlm.nih.gov/pubmed/19647123

FROM FULL TEXT:

"Evidence suggests that the endocannabinoid system may be dysregulated in a number of cancers (summarized in Table 18.1). Indeed, both AEA and 2-arachidonyl glycerol (2-AG) have been shown to be increased in human colorectal adenomatous polyps and carcinomas compared to normal colorectal mucosa (Ligresti et al., 2003), suggesting that these endocannabinoids increase when passing from normal to transformed mucosa. No consistent differences were observed in the expression levels of Cb1, Cb2, or FAAH as assessed by both RT-PCR and immunoblotting between normal and colorectal cancer tissue (Ligresti et al., 2003). Similarly, AEA levels were enhanced by 17-fold in glioblastomas whereas meningiomas were characterized by a massively enhanced level of 2-AG (Petersen et al., 2005). Coupled with these changes was a 60% reduction in the enzyme activities of the AEA degradation enzymes, N-acylphosphotidylethanolamine-hydrolyzing phospholipase D and fatty acid amide hydrolase in the glioblastoma tissue and an enhanced in vitro conversion of phosphotidyl choline to monoacyl glycerol in the meningioma tissue (Petersen et al., 2005). Similarly, the levels of AEA and 2-AG were found to be increased in human pituitary adenomas compared to normal pituitary gland (Pagotto et al., 2001). Moreover, endocannabinoid content in the different pituitary adenomas correlated with the presence of Cb1, being elevated in the tumoral samples positive for Cb1 and lower in the samples in which no or low levels of Cb1 were found (Pagotto et al., 2001). In another study, the levels of AEA were found to differ depending upon the source of the tumor (Schmid et al., 2002). For example, AEA was increased in prostate carcinoma, endometrial sarcoma, and thigh histiocytoma, with no change in ileum lymphoma, and bladder carcinoma and a significant decrease in stomach carcinoma (Schmidet al., 2002). Furthermore, the cannabinoid receptor system has also been shown to be altered during the carcinogenic process. Indeed, in Mantle cell lymphoma and prostate cancer cells, both Cb1 and Cb2 are upregulated compared to nonmalignant tissue (Ek et al., 2002; Islam et al., 2003; Sarfaraz et al., 2005), whereas in acute myeloid leukemia, only Cb2 is upregulated (Alberich Jorda et al., 2004). In conclusion, the endocannabinoid system exerts a myriad of effects on tumor cell growth, progression, angiogenesis, and migration. With a notable few exceptions, targeting the endocannabinoid system with agents that activate cannabinoid receptors or increase the endogenous levels of AEA may prove to have therapeutic benefit in the treatment of various cancers. Further studies into the downstream consequences of AEA treatment are required and may illuminate other potential therapeutic targets."

Complete Study Links:

https://www.ncbi.nlm.nih.gov/pmc/articles/PMC2791688/
https://www.ncbi.nlm.nih.gov/pmc/articles/PMC2791688/pdf/nihms16018
0.pdf

Cannabinoid action induces autophagy-mediated cell death through stimulation of ER stress in human glioma cells.

Journal of Clinical Investigation.

María Salazar,[1,2] Arkaitz Carracedo,[1] Íñigo J. Salanueva,[1] Sonia Hernández-Tiedra,[1] Mar Lorente,[1,2]

Ainara Egia,[1] Patricia Vázquez,[3] Cristina Blázquez,[1,2] Sofía Torres,[1] Stephane García,[4]

Jonathan Nowak,[4] Gian María Fimia,[5] Mauro Piacentini,[5] Francesco Cecconi,[6] Pier Paolo Pandolfi,[7]

Luis González-Feria,[8] Juan L. Iovanna,[4] Manuel Guzmán,[1,2] Patricia Boya,[3] and Guillermo Velasco[1,2]

[1]Department of Biochemistry and Molecular Biology I, School of Biology, Complutense University, Madrid, Spain.

[2] Centro de Investigación Biomédica en Red sobre Enfermedades Neurodegenerativas (CIBERNED), Madrid, Spain.

[3] 3D Lab (Development, Differentiation, and Degeneration), Department of Cellular and Molecular Physiopathology, Centro de Investigaciones Biológicas, Consejo Superior de Investigaciones Científicas (CSIC), Madrid, Spain.

[4] INSERM U624, Campus de Luminy, Marseille, France.

[5] National Institute for Infectious Diseases, IRCCS "L. Spallanzani," Rome, Italy.

[6] Laboratory of Molecular Neuroembryology, IRCCS Fondazione Santa Lucia and Department of Biology, University of Rome "Tor Vergata," Rome, Italy.

[7] Cancer Genetics Program, Beth Israel Deaconess Cancer Center and Department of Medicine, Beth Israel Deaconess Medical Center, Harvard Medical School, Boston, Massachusetts, USA. 8Department of Neurosurgery, University Hospital, Tenerife, Spain.

Abstract

Autophagy can promote cell survival or cell death, but the molecular basis underlying its dual role in cancer remains obscure. Here we demonstrate that delta(9)-tetrahydrocannabinol (THC), the main active component of marijuana, induces human glioma cell death through stimulation of autophagy. Our data indicate that THC induced ceramide accumulation and eukaryotic translation initiation factor 2alpha (eIF2alpha) phosphorylation and thereby activated an ER stress response that promoted autophagy via tribbles homolog

3-dependent (TRB3-dependent) inhibition of the Akt/mammalian target of rapamycin complex 1 (mTORC1) axis. We also showed that autophagy is upstream of apoptosis in cannabinoid-induced human and mouse cancer cell death and that activation of this pathway was necessary for the antitumor action of cannabinoids in vivo. These findings describe a mechanism by which THC can promote the autophagic death of human and mouse cancer cells and provide evidence that cannabinoid administration may be an effective therapeutic strategy for targeting human cancers.

PubMed Link: https://www.ncbi.nlm.nih.gov/pubmed/19425170

FROM FULL TEXT:
"In this study we show that cannabinoids, a new family of potential antitumoral agents, induce autophagy of cancer cells and that this process mediates the cell death–promoting activity of these compounds. Several observations strongly support this idea: (a) THC induced autophagy and cell death in different types of cancer cells but not in nontransformed astrocytes, which are resistant to cannabinoid killing action, (b) pharmacological or genetic inhibition of autophagy prevented THC-induced cell death, (c) autophagydeficient tumors were resistant to THC growth-inhibiting action, and (d) THC administration activated the autophagic cell death pathway in 3 different models of tumor xenografts as well as in 2 human tumor samples. Depending on the cellular context and the strength and duration of the triggering stimulus, autophagy is involved in the promotion or inhibition of cancer cell survival (4, 5, 24, 25). However, the molecular bases of this dual role of autophagy in cancer remain unknown."

Complete Study Links:
https://www.ncbi.nlm.nih.gov/pmc/articles/PMC2673842/
https://www.ncbi.nlm.nih.gov/pmc/articles/PMC2673842/pdf/JCI37948.pdf

Endocannabinoid system modulation in cancer biology and therapy.
Pharmacological Research.

Pisanti S, Bifulco M.
Department of Pharmaceutical Sciences, University of Salerno, Italy.

Abstract
The discovery of the endocannabinoid system and the recognition of its potential impact in a plethora of pathological conditions, led to the development of therapeutic agents related to either the stimulation or antagonism of CB1 and CB2 cannabinoid receptors, the majority of which are actually tested in preclinical studies for the pharmacotherapy of several diseases. Endocannabinoid-related agents have been reported to affect multiple signaling pathways and biological processes involved in the development of cancer, displaying an interesting anti-proliferative, pro-apoptotic, anti-angiogenic and anti-metastatic activity both in vitro and in vivo in several models of cancer. Emerging evidence

suggests that agonists of cannabinoid receptors, which share the useful property to discern between tumor cells and their non-transformed counterparts, could represent novel tumor-selective tools to treat cancer in addition to their already exploited use as palliative drugs to treat chemotherapy-induced nausea, pain and anorexia/weight loss in cancer patients. The aim of this review is to evidence and update the recent emerging knowledge about the role of the endocannabinoid system in cancer biology and the potentiality of its modulation in cancer therapy.

PubMed Link: https://www.ncbi.nlm.nih.gov/pubmed/19559362

Cannabinoid receptor ligands as potential anticancer agents--high hopes for new therapies?
Journal of Pharmacy and Pharmacology.

Oesch S, Gertsch J.
University Children's Hospital Divisions of Clinical Chemistry and Oncology, University of Zürich, Switzerland.

Abstract
OBJECTIVES:
The endocannabinoid system is an endogenous lipid signalling network comprising arachidonic-acid-derived ligands, cannabinoid (CB) receptors, transporters and endocannabinoid degrading enzymes. The CB(1) receptor is predominantly expressed in neurons but is also co-expressed with the CB(2) receptor in peripheral tissues. In recent years, CB receptor ligands, including Delta(9)-tetrahydrocannabinol, have been proposed as potential anticancer agents.
KEY FINDINGS:
This review critically discusses the pharmacology of CB receptor activation as a novel therapeutic anticancer strategy in terms of ligand selectivity, tissue specificity and potency. Intriguingly, antitumour effects mediated by cannabinoids are not confined to inhibition of cancer cell proliferation; cannabinoids also reduce angiogenesis, cell migration and metastasis, inhibit carcinogenesis and attenuate inflammatory processes. In the last decade several new selective CB(1) and CB(2) receptor agents have been described, but most studies in the area of cancer research have used non-selective CB ligands. Moreover, many of these ligands exert prominent CB receptor-independent pharmacological effects, such as activation of the G-protein-coupled receptor GPR55, peroxisome proliferator-activated receptor gamma and the transient receptor potential vanilloid channels.
SUMMARY:
The role of the endocannabinoid system in tumourigenesis is still poorly understood and the molecular mechanisms of cannabinoid anticancer action need to be elucidated. The development of CB(2)-selective anticancer agents could be advantageous in light of the unwanted central effects exerted by CB(1) receptor ligands. Probably the most interesting question is whether cannabinoids could be useful in chemoprevention or in combination with established chemotherapeutic agents.

PubMed Link: https://www.ncbi.nlm.nih.gov/pubmed/19589225

The CB1/CB2 receptor agonist WIN-55,212-2 reduces viability of human Kaposi's sarcoma cells in vitro.

European Journal of Pharmacology.

Luca T, Di Benedetto G, Scuderi MR, Palumbo M,
Clementi S, Bernardini R, Cantarella G.
Department of Experimental and Clinical Pharmacology, University of
Catania School of Medicine, Catania, Italy.

Abstract
Kaposi's sarcoma is a highly vascularized mesenchymal neoplasm arising with multiple lesions of the skin. Endogenous cannabinoids have been shown to inhibit proliferation of a wide spectrum of tumor cells. We studied the effects of cannabinoids on human Kaposi's sarcoma cell proliferation in vitro. To do so, we first investigated the presence of the cannabinoid receptors CB(1) and CB(2) mRNAs in the human Kaposi's sarcoma cell line KS-IMM by RT-PCR and, subsequently, the effects of the mixed CB(1)/CB(2) agonist WIN-55,212-2 (WIN) on cell proliferation in vitro. WIN showed antimitogenic effects on Kaposi's sarcoma cells. Western blot analysis of Kaposi's sarcoma lysates suggested that WIN treatment induced activation of both caspase-3 and -6, as well as increased phospho-rylation of the stress kinase p38 and JNK, along with transient phosphorylation of ERK(1/2). To better characterize the involvement of each single CB receptor in cannabi-noid-induced cell death, we incubated Kaposi's sarcoma cells with different selective cannabinoid receptor agonists, respectively ACEA (CB(1)) and JWH-133 (CB(2)). None of the agonists was able to induce KS-IMM cell apoptosis. Moreover, we co-incubated Kaposi's sarcoma cells with WIN-55,212-2 and either the CB(1) receptor antagonist AM251, the CB(2) receptor antagonist AM630, or a combination of both substances. The CB(2) receptor antagonist AM630 was able to significantly increase survival of Kaposi's sarcoma cells treated with WIN. In view of the antiproliferative effects of cannabinoids on KS-IMM cells, one could envision the cannabinoid system as a potential target for pharmacological treatment of Kaposi's sarcoma.

PubMed Link: https://www.ncbi.nlm.nih.gov/pubmed/19539619

FROM FULL TEXT:

"Here we show that the Kaposis's sarcoma cell line KS-IMM, which expresses both CB1 and CB2 cannabinoid receptors, respond to agonists with decreased proliferation. In fact, the mixed CB1/CB2 agonist WIN-55,212-2 can induce Kaposi's sarcoma cell death after 72 h of treatment. Morphological changes of Kaposi's sarcoma cells and bis-benzimide nuclear staining indicates that such cannabinoid-induced death was of the apoptotic type."

Complete Study Links:
http://www.sciencedirect.com/science/article/pii/S0014299909005159

Cannabinoid receptor 1 is a potential drug target for treatment of translocation-positive rhabdomyosarcoma.

Molecular Cancer Theraputics.

Oesch S, Walter D, Wachtel M, Pretre K, Salazar M, Guzmán M, Velasco G, Schäfer BW.

Department of Oncology, University Children's Hospital, Zurich, Switzerland.

Abstract

Gene expression profiling has revealed that the gene coding for cannabinoid receptor 1 (CB1) is highly up-regulated in rhabdomyosarcoma biopsies bearing the typical chromosomal translocations PAX3/FKHR or PAX7/FKHR. Because cannabinoid receptor agonists are capable of reducing proliferation and inducing apoptosis in diverse cancer cells such as glioma, breast cancer, and melanoma, we evaluated whether CB1 is a potential drug target in rhabdomyosarcoma. Our study shows that treatment with the cannabinoid receptor agonists HU210 and Delta(9)-tetrahydrocannabinol lowers the viability of translocation-positive rhabdomyosarcoma cells through the induction of apoptosis. This effect relies on inhibition of AKT signaling and induction of the stress-associated transcription factor p8 because small interfering RNA-mediated down-regulation of p8 rescued cell viability upon cannabinoid treatment. Finally, treatment of xenografts with HU210 led to a significant suppression of tumor growth in vivo. These results support the notion that cannabinoid receptor agonists could represent a novel targeted approach for treatment of translocation-positive rhabdomyosarcoma.

PubMed Link: https://www.ncbi.nlm.nih.gov/pubmed/19509271

FROM FULL TEXT:

"Rhabdomyosarcoma (RMS) is the most common soft-tissue sarcoma in children, representing 5% to 8% of all childhood malignancies (1). It is believed to originate from muscle precursor cells and histology recognizes two major subtypes: The embryonal subtype (eRMS) accounts for 60% of RMS cases and has a rather good prognosis (2). The alveolar subtype (2) is less frequent, more aggressive, usually presents with metastasis, and is thus associated with rather poor treatment outcome.

In vitro, cannabinoid receptor agonists HU210, THC, and Met-F-AEA exerted an antiproliferative and proapoptotic action on tposRMS cells through activation of the CB1 receptor. The specificity of this effect for CB1 was shown by two means: First, the cell viability in fibroblasts or tnegRMS control cell lines, which express only low levels of CB1, is not affected. Second, the CB1-specific antagonist AM251 was able to significantly reduce apoptosis and partially restore cell viability. TposRMS cells were most sensitive to submicromolar concentrations of HU210, THC, and Met-F-AEA, and comparable with those observed in other cancer cells such as pancreatic cancer (20), breast cancer (22), or colon cancer (27) cells.

In summary, our results support and extend the previously shown antitumor activities of cannabinoid receptor agonists by showing proapoptotic effects of HU210, THC, and Met-F-AEA on tposRMS cells in vitro and, for the first time, show that HU210 has tumor growth inhibiting properties in vivo. This could represent one possible novel treatment strategy that might improve outcome in this pediatric tumor."

Complete Study Links:
http://mct.aacrjournals.org/content/8/7/1838.long
http://mct.aacrjournals.org/content/molcanther/8/7/1838.full.pdf

Cannabinoids in intestinal inflammation and cancer.
Pharmacological Research.

Izzo AA, Camilleri M.
Department of Experimental Pharmacology, University of Naples Federico II and Endocannabinoid Research Group, Naples, Italy.

Abstract
Emerging evidence suggests that cannabinoids may exert beneficial effects in intestinal inflammation and cancer. Adaptive changes of the endocannabinoid system have been observed in intestinal biopsies from patients with inflammatory bowel disease and colon cancer. Studies on epithelial cells have shown that cannabinoids exert antiproliferative, antimetastatic and apoptotic effects as well as reducing cytokine release and promoting wound healing. In vivo, cannabinoids - via direct or indirect activation of CB(1) and/or CB(2) receptors - exert protective effects in well-established models of intestinal inflammation and colon cancer. Pharmacological elevation of endocannabinoid levels may be a promising strategy to counteract intestinal inflammation and colon cancer.

PubMed Link: https://www.ncbi.nlm.nih.gov/pubmed/19442536

Cannabidiol inhibits cancer cell invasion via upregulation of tissue inhibitor of matrix metalloproteinases-1.

Biochem Pharmacol.

Ramer R, Merkord J, Rohde H, Hinz B.
Institute of Toxicology and Pharmacology, University of Rostock, Schillingallee 70, D-18057 Rostock, Germany.

Abstract (edited)

"Although cannabinoids exhibit a broad variety of anticarcinogenic effects, their potential use in cancer therapy is limited by their psychoactive effects. Here we evaluated the impact of cannabidiol, a plant-derived non-psychoactive cannabinoid, on cancer cell invasion.... Altogether, these findings provide a novel mechanism underlying the anti-invasive action of cannabidiol and imply its use as a therapeutic option for the treatment of highly invasive cancers."

PubMed Link: https://www.ncbi.nlm.nih.gov/pubmed/19914218

Synthetic cannabinoid receptor agonists inhibit tumor growth and metastasis of breast cancer.

Molecular Cancer Theraputics.

Qamri Z, Preet A, Nasser MW, Bass CE, Leone G, Barsky SH, Ganju RK.
Department of Pathology, Ohio State University Medical Center, Columbus, OH, USA.

Abstract

Cannabinoids have been reported to possess antitumorogenic activity. Not much is known, however, about the effects and mechanism of action of synthetic nonpsychotic cannabinoids on breast cancer growth and metastasis. We have shown that the cannabinoid receptors CB1 and CB2 are overexpressed in primary human breast tumors compared with normal breast tissue. We have also observed that the breast cancer cell lines MDA-MB231, MDA-MB231-luc, and MDA-MB468 express CB1 and CB2 receptors. Furthermore, we have shown that the CB2 synthetic agonist JWH-133 and the CB1 and CB2 agonist WIN-55,212-2 inhibit cell proliferation and migration under in vitro conditions. These results were confirmed in vivo in various mouse model systems. Mice treated with JWH-133 or WIN-55,212-2 showed a 40% to 50% reduction in tumor growth and a 65% to 80% reduction in lung metastasis. These effects were reversed by CB1 and CB2 antagonists AM 251 and SR144528, respectively, suggesting involvement of CB1 and CB2 receptors. In addition, the CB2 agonist JWH-133 was shown to delay and reduce mammary gland tumors in the polyoma middle T oncoprotein (PyMT) transgenic mouse model system. Upon further elucidation, we observed that JWH-133 and WIN-55,212-2 mediate the breast tumor-suppressive effects via a coordinated regulation of cyclooxygenase-2/prostaglandin E2 signaling pathways and induction of apoptosis. These results indicate that CB1 and CB2 receptors could be used to develop novel therapeutic strategies against breast cancer growth and metastasis.

PubMed Link: https://www.ncbi.nlm.nih.gov/pubmed/19887554

FROM FULL TEXT:

Despite advances in the early detection of breast cancer, about 30% of patients with early stage have recurrent disease (1). Systemic treatment of breast cancer includes cytotoxic, hormonal, and immunotherapeutic agents, which are active at the beginning of therapy in 90% of primary breast cancers and 50% of metastases. After a variable period of time, however, progression occurs and multidrug resistance is observed (2–5). Thus, further studies are necessary to determine novel targets and mechanism-based agents with increased efficacy and low toxicity for prevention and treatment of this disease. In the present study, therefore, we analyzed the effects of synthetic cannabinoids on breast cancer cells. Currently, there are three general types of cannabinoids: phytocannabinoids, and endogenous and synthetic cannabinoids. These function through two different specific cell surface G-protein coupled receptors, CB1 and CB2 (6, 7). The CB1 receptor is predominantly expressed in the central nervous system, whereas the CB2 receptor is expressed by immune cells. Cannabinoid receptors have been reported to be overexpressed in prostate, skin, and hepatocellular carcinoma (8–10). Experimental evidence has shown that cannabinoids inhibit the growth of tumor xenograft in mice (8, 11–14). Cannabinoids have been shown to inhibit tumor angiogenesis and directly induce apoptosis or cell cycle arrest in neoplastic cells (8, 11–14). Although these studies point to the potential application of cannabinoids as antitumor agents in various human cancer cells, not much is known about the molecular mechanism of cannabinoid-mediated antimetastatic and tumurogenic effects.

Complete Study Links:

http://mct.aacrjournals.org/content/8/11/3117.long
http://mct.aacrjournals.org/content/8/11/3117.full-text.pdf

2010

The dual effects of delta(9)-tetrahydrocannabinol on cholangiocarcinoma cells: anti-invasion activity at low concentration and apoptosis induction at high concentration.

Cancer Investigation.

Leelawat S, Leelawat K, Narong S, Matangkasombut O.
Faculty of Pharmacy, Rangsit University, Patumthani, Thailand.

Abstract

Currently, only gemcitabine plus platinum demonstrates the considerable activity for cholangiocarcinoma. The anticancer effect of Delta (9)-tetrahydrocannabinol (THC), the principal active component of cannabinoids has been demonstrated in various kinds of cancers. We therefore evaluate the antitumor effects of THC on cholangiocarcinoma cells.

Both cholangiocarcinoma cell lines and surgical specimens from cholangiocarcinoma patients expressed cannabinoid receptors. THC inhibited cell proliferation, migration and invasion, and induced cell apoptosis. THC also decreased actin polymerization and reduced tumor cell survival in anoikis assay. pMEK1/2 and pAkt demonstrated the lower extent than untreated cells. Consequently, THC is potentially used to retard cholangiocarcinoma cell growth and metastasis.

PubMed Link: https://www.ncbi.nlm.nih.gov/pubmed/19916793

Antitumorigenic effects of cannabinoids beyond apoptosis.

Journal of Pharmacology and Experimental Theraputics

Freimuth N, Ramer R, Hinz B.
Institute of Toxicology and Pharmacology, University of Rostock, Rostock, Germany.

Abstract

According to the World Health Organization, the cases of death caused by cancer will have been doubled until the year 2030. By 2010, cancer is expected to be the number one cause of death. Therefore, it is necessary to explore novel approaches for the treatment of cancer. Over past years, the antitumorigenic effects of cannabinoids have emerged as an exciting field in cancer research. Apart from their proapoptotic and antiproliferative action, recent research has shown that cannabinoids may likewise affect tumor cell angiogenesis, migration, invasion, adhesion, and metastasization. This review will summarize the data concerning the influence of cannabinoids on these locomotive processes beyond modulation of cancer cell apoptosis and proliferation. The findings discussed here provide a new perspective on the antitumorigenic potential of cannabinoids.

PubMed Link: https://www.ncbi.nlm.nih.gov/pubmed/19889794

FROM FULL TEXT:

"Cannabinoids are currently used in cancer patients to palliate wasting, emesis, and pain. In addition, evidence has been accumulated over the last decade to suggest that these compounds could also be useful for the inhibition of tumor cell growth by modulating several survival pathways. Although anticancer effects of cannabinoids were shown as early as 1975 in Lewis lung carcinoma (Munson et al., 1975), interest in anticarcinogenic properties of these compounds was even renewed after the discovery of the cannabinoid system and the cloning of specific Gi/o-coupled cannabinoid receptors CB1 and CB2 (De Petrocellis et al., 1998; for review, see also Howlett et al., 2002; Abood, 2005). Recent investigations have shown that besides its well known antiapoptotic and antiproliferative action, cannabinoids may also confer antiangiogenic, antimigrative, antiadhesive, anti-invasive, and antimetastatic properties by pathways including activation of both cannabinoid receptors as well as TRPV1. Although a limited number of studies have been published addressing the underlying mechanisms, the currently avail-

148

able results indicate that the modulation of several components of signal transduction pathways, including Src, nuclear factor B, ERK1/2, HIF-1, Akt, and modulation of the expression as well as that of the enzymatic action of proteins of the MMP family, EGF, VEGF, IgSF CAMs, and FAK, by cannabinoids might support beneficial effects on tumor cell locomotion and spreading. Based on these facts, evidence is emerging to suggest that cannabinoids are potent inhibitors of both cancer growth and spreading. Because cannabinoids are usually well tolerated and do not develop the toxic effects of conventional chemotherapeutics, more preclinical studies are warranted to investigate a potential utility of these substances as anticancer therapeutics."

Complete Study Links:
http://jpet.aspetjournals.org/content/332/2/336.long
http://jpet.aspetjournals.org/content/jpet/332/2/336.full.pdf

Cannabidiol enhances the inhibitory effects of delta9-tetrahydrocannabinol on human glioblastoma cell proliferation and survival.

Molecular Cancer Theraputics.

Marcu JP, Christian RT, Lau D, Zielinski AJ, Horowitz MP, Lee J, Pakdel A, Allison J, Limbad C, Moore DH, Yount GL, Desprez PY, McAllister SD. California Pacific Medical Center Research Institute, San Francisco, California, USA.

Abstract

The cannabinoid 1 (CB(1)) and cannabinoid 2 (CB(2)) receptor agonist Delta(9)-tetrahydrocannabinol (THC) has been shown to be a broad-range inhibitor of cancer in culture and in vivo, and is currently being used in a clinical trial for the treatment of glioblastoma. It has been suggested that other plant-derived cannabinoids, which do not interact efficiently with CB(1) and CB(2) receptors, can modulate the actions of Delta(9)-THC. There are conflicting reports, however, as to what extent other cannabinoids can modulate Delta(9)-THC activity, and most importantly, it is not clear whether other cannabinoid compounds can either potentiate or inhibit the actions of Delta(9)-THC. We therefore tested cannabidiol, the second most abundant plant-derived cannabinoid, in combination with Delta(9)-THC. In the U251 and SF126 glioblastoma cell lines, Delta(9)-THC and cannabidiol acted synergistically to inhibit cell proliferation. The treatment of glioblastoma cells with both compounds led to significant modulations of the cell cycle and induction of reactive oxygen species and apoptosis as well as specific modulations of extracellular signal-regulated kinase and caspase activities. These specific changes were not observed with either compound individually, indicating that the signal transduction pathways affected by the combination treatment were unique. Our results suggest that the addition of cannabidiol to Delta(9)-THC may improve the overall effectiveness of Delta(9)-THC in the treatment of glioblastoma in cancer patients.

PubMed Link: https://www.ncbi.nlm.nih.gov/pubmed/20053780

FROM FULL TEXT:

"There are conflicting reports as to what extent other cannabinoids can modulate the activity of Δ9-THC, and it has been suggested that nonpsychoactive cannabinoids can either potentiate or inhibit the actions of Δ9-THC (17–20). Cooperative effects have also been observed with endogenous cannabinoids (21). The potential benefits of using a cannabinoid-based medicine comprising multiple cannabinoids has been a driving force in recent human clinical trials (20, 22, 23). Investigations have shown that nonpyschoactive cannabinoids can alter the physiologic response to Δ9-THC, potentially by altering its metabolism (17–19, 24, 25). However, no investigation to date has provided the molecular mechanisms to explain how cannabinoids, acting through distinct pathways, could converge onto a shared pathway resulting in a modulation of activity unique to the combination. In this study, we sought to determine whether cannabidiol, the plant-derived cannabinoid, would modulate the ability of Δ9-THC to inhibit glioblastoma cell proliferation and survival. We found that cannabidiol enhanced the ability of Δ9-THC to inhibit glioblastoma cell growth and induce apoptosis. The molecular mechanisms associated with these specific effects are presented."

Complete Study Links:

http://mct.aacrjournals.org/content/9/1/180.long
http://mct.aacrjournals.org/content/molcanther/9/1/180.full.pdf

Effects of anandamide on polyamine levels and cell growth in human colon cancer cells.

Anticancer Research.

Linsalata M, Notarnicola M, Tutino V, Bifulco M,
Santoro A, Laezza C, Messa C, Orlando A, Caruso MG.
Laboratory of Biochemistry, National Institute for Digestive Diseases, Via Turi 27, Castellana Grotte, Bari, Italy.

Abstract

BACKGROUND:

Anandamide (AEA) is an endogenous agonist for cannabinoid receptor CB1-R and seems to be involved in the control of cancer growth. Polyamines are compounds that play an important role in cell proliferation and differentiation. Our aim was to investigate the effect of AEA on the polyamine levels (putrescine, spermidine and spermine) and cell growth of three human colon cancer cell lines, positive for CB1-R.

MATERIALS AND METHODS:

After AEA treatment of DLD-1, HT-29 and SW620 cells, polyamine analysis was performed by high-performance liquid chromatography (HPLC) and cell growth was measured by 3-(4,5 di-methylthiazol-2-yl)-2,5-diphenyltetrazolium bromide (MTT) test. CB1 gene expression was determined using reverse transcription and polymerase chain reaction (RT-PCR).

RESULTS:

AEA significantly reduced polyamine levels and cell proliferation dose-dependently when the tested cell lines were exposed for 24 h and 48 h. This inhibitory effect was mediated by CB1-R, since SR 1411716A, a selective CB-1 receptor antagonist, was able to entirely antagonize the effect of AEA. CB1-R mRNA levels were enhanced after AEA treatment in DLD-1 cells, whereas no induction was found in HT-29 and SW620 cells.

CONCLUSION:

It appears that mechanisms by which AEA may affect growth of colon cancer cells involve a decrease in cell proliferation rate by reducing the polyamine levels.

PubMed Link: https://www.ncbi.nlm.nih.gov/pubmed/20682986

Cannabinoids reduce ErbB2-driven breast cancer progression through Akt inhibition.

Molecular Cancer.

Caffarel MM, Andradas C, Mira E, Pérez-Gómez E, Cerutti C, Moreno-Bueno G, Flores JM, García-Real I, Palacios J, Mañes S, Guzmán M, Sánchez C.
Dept, Biochemistry and Molecular Biology I, School of Biology, Complutense University, Madrid, Spain.

Abstract

BACKGROUND:

ErbB2-positive breast cancer is characterized by highly aggressive phenotypes and reduced responsiveness to standard therapies. Although specific ErbB2-targeted therapies have been designed, only a small percentage of patients respond to these treatments and most of them eventually relapse. The existence of this population of particularly aggressive and non-responding or relapsing patients urges the search for novel therapies. The purpose of this study was to determine whether cannabinoids might constitute a new therapeutic tool for the treatment of ErbB2-positive breast tumors. We analyzed their antitumor potential in a well established and clinically relevant model of ErbB2-driven metastatic breast cancer: the MMTV-neu mouse. We also analyzed the expression of cannabinoid targets in a series of 87 human breast tumors.

RESULTS:

Our results show that both Delta9-tetrahydrocannabinol, the most abundant and potent cannabinoid in marijuana, and JWH-133, a non-psychotropic CB2 receptor-selective agonist, reduce tumor growth, tumor number, and the amount/severity of lung metastases in MMTV-neu mice. Histological analyses of the tumors revealed that cannabinoids inhibit cancer cell proliferation, induce cancer cell apoptosis, and impair tumor angiogenesis. Cannabinoid antitumoral action relies, at least partially, on the inhibition of the pro-tumorigenic Akt pathway. We also found that 91% of ErbB2-positive tumors express the non-psychotropic cannabinoid receptor CB2.

CONCLUSIONS:

Taken together, these results provide a strong preclinical evidence for the use of cannabinoid-based therapies for the management of ErbB2-positive breast cancer.

PubMed Link: https://www.ncbi.nlm.nih.gov/pubmed/20649976

FROM FULL TEXT:

"Breast cancer represents approximately 30% of newly diagnosed cancers each year.... The therapeutic potential of cannabinoids, the active compounds of marijuana and their derivatives, has been known for centuries. There is increasing evidence supporting that they might be beneficial in various pathological contexts such as pain, inflammation, eating disorders, and brain damage, amongst others [5,6]. Cannabinoids exert most of their actions by binding to and activating specific G protein-coupled receptors. To date, two cannabinoid receptors, namely CB1 and CB2, have been cloned and characterized from mammalian tissues, the main difference between them being their tissue expression pattern. Thus, while CB1 receptors are ubiquitously located, with their highest presence found in the central nervous system, CB2 receptor expression is mostly restricted to particular elements of the immune system [5,6]. During the last decade, evidence has accumulated suggesting that cannabinoids might be useful for the treatment of cancer. These compounds exert anti-proliferative, pro-apoptotic, anti-angiogenic, and anti-invasive effects in different cell-culture and animal models of cancer [7,8]."

Complete Study Links:

https://molecular-cancer.biomedcentral.com/articles/10.1186/1476-4598-9-196

https://www.ncbi.nlm.nih.gov/pmc/articles/PMC2917429/

https://www.ncbi.nlm.nih.gov/pmc/articles/PMC2917429/pdf/1476-4598-9-196.pdf

Cannabinoids inhibit cellular respiration of human oral cancer cells.

Pharmacology.

Whyte DA, Al-Hammadi S, Balhaj G, Brown OM, Penefsky HS, Souid AK. Department of Pediatricsy, State University of New York, Upstate Medical University, Syracuse, NY, USA.

Abstract

BACKGROUND AND PURPOSE:

The primary cannabinoids, Delta(9)-tetrahydrocannabinol (Delta(9)-THC) and Delta(8)-tetrahydrocannabinol (Delta(8)-THC) are known to disturb the mitochondrial function and possess antitumor activities. These observations prompted us to investigate their effects on the mitochondrial O(2) consumption in human oral cancer cells (Tu183). This epithelial cell line overexpresses bcl-2 and is highly resistant to anticancer drugs.

EXPERIMENTAL APPROACH:

A phosphorescence analyzer that measures the time-dependence of O(2) concentration in cellular or mitochondrial suspensions was used for this purpose.

KEY RESULTS:

A rapid decline in the rate of respiration was observed when Delta(9)-THC or Delta(8)-THC was added to the cells. The inhibition was concentration-dependent, and Delta(9)-THC was the more potent of the two compounds. Anandamide (an endocannabinoid) was ineffective; suggesting the effects of Delta(9)-THC and Delta(8)-THC were not mediated by the cannabinoidreceptors. Inhibition of O(2) consumption by cyanide confirmed the oxidations occurred in the mitochondrial respiratory chain. Delta(9)-THC inhibited the respiration of isolated mitochondria from beef heart.

CONCLUSIONS AND IMPLICATIONS:

These results show the cannabinoids are potent inhibitors of Tu183 cellular respiration and are toxic to this highly malignant tumor.

PubMed Link: https://www.ncbi.nlm.nih.gov/pubmed/20516734

FROM FULL TEXT:

"Oral squamous cell carcinoma is the 6th most common malignancy. This cancer is responsible for the death of over 8,000 patients per year in the US [20]. The tumor remains one of the hardest to treat, not only because of its poor response to therapy, but also due to physical complications posed by the surgery. Moreover, oral cancer cells (e.g., Tu183 cells) are known to adapt genetic changes that block cell death.

Our results show that cannabinoids (especially ^9-THC) are potent inhibitors of Tul83 cell respiration (fig. 1). Furthermore, the effect of ^9-THC is immediate (fig.1c) and more potent than observed with commonly used anticancer drugs (fig.3). On the other hand, anandamide (an endocannabinoid) is ineffective, suggesting the effects of ^9-THC and ^8-THC are not mediated through cannabinoid receptors."

Complete Study Link:

https://www.karger.com/Article/Abstract/312686

Effect of a synthetic cannabinoid agonist on the proliferation and invasion of gastric cancer cells.

J Cell Biochem.

Xian XS, Park H, Cho YK, Lee IS, Kim SW, Choi MG, Chung IS, Han KH, Park JM.

Division of Gastroenterology, Department of Internal Medicine, College of Medicine, The Catholic University of Korea, Seoul, Korea.

Abstract

Although cannabinoids are associated with antineoplastic activity in a number of cancer cell types, the effect in gastric cancer cells has not been clarified. In the present study, we investigated the effects of a cannabinoid agonist on gastric cancer cell proliferation and invasion. The cannabinoid agonist WIN 55,212-2 inhibited the proliferation of human gastric cancer cells in a dose-dependent manner and that this effect was mediated partially by the CB(1) receptor. We also found that WIN 55,212-2 induced apoptosis and down-regulation of the phospho-AKT expression in human gastric cancer cells. Furthermore, WIN 55,212-2 treatment inhibited the invasion of gastric cancer cells, and down-regulated the expression of MMP-2 and VEGF-A through the cannabinoid receptors. Our results open the possibilities in using cannabinoids as a new gastric cancer therapy.

PubMed Link: https://www.ncbi.nlm.nih.gov/pubmed/20336665

Opposing actions of endocannabinoids on cholangiocarcinoma growth is via the differential activation of Notch signaling.

Experimental Cell Research.

Frampton G, Coufal M, Li H, Ramirez J, DeMorrow S.
Department of Internal Medicine, Texas A&M Health Science Center College of Medicine, Temple, TX, USA.

Abstract (edited):
"The development of novel therapeutic strategies aimed at modulating the endocannabinoid system or mimicking the mode of action of AEA on Notch signaling pathways would prove beneficial for cholangiocarcinoma management."

PubMed Link: https://www.ncbi.nlm.nih.gov/pubmed/20347808

Complete Study Links:

https://www.ncbi.nlm.nih.gov/pmc/articles/PMC2872061/
https://www.ncbi.nlm.nih.gov/pmc/articles/PMC2872061/pdf/nihms19288 8.pdf

Cannabinoids attenuate cancer pain and proliferation in a mouse model.

Neuroscience Letters.

Saghafi N, Lam DK, Schmidt BL.Author information
UCSF School of Dentistry, University of California San Francisco, United States.

Abstract
We investigated the effects of cannabinoid receptor agonists on (1) oral cancer cell viability in vitro and (2) oral cancer pain and tumor growth in a mouse cancer model. We utilized immunohistochemistry and Western blot to show that human oral cancer cells express CBr1 and CBr2. When treated with WIN55,212-2 (non-selective), ACEA (CBr1-selective) or AM1241 (CBr2-selective) agonists in vitro, oral cancer cell proliferation was significantly attenuated in a dose-dependent manner. In vivo, systemic administration (0.013M) of WIN55,212-2, ACEA, or AM1241 significantly attenuated cancer-induced mechanical allodynia. Tumor growth was also significantly attenuated with systemic AM1241 administration. Our findings suggest a direct role for cannabinoid mechanisms in oral cancer pain and proliferation. The systemic administration of cannabinoid receptor agonists may have important therapeutic implications wherein cannabinoid receptor agonists may reduce morbidity and mortality of oral cancer.

PubMed Link: https://www.ncbi.nlm.nih.gov/pubmed/21094209

FROM FULL TEXT:

"Oral cancer represents 3% of all cancers and its overall survival rate of 50% places it among the worst of all cancers [18,31]. Approximately 50,000 new cases of head and neck cancer are diagnosed each year in the United States [11]. Therefore, there is a concerted effort to discover its cure. Many different agents are currently being investigated for their palliative or anti-proliferative properties on cancer. Of particular interest are cannabinoids, a group of chemicals found in Cannabis sativa Linnaeus plant and their derivatives [2,8,27]. The two widely recognized cannabinoid receptors, CBr1 and CBr2, are G-protein-coupled receptors [22]. CBr1 is expressed mainly in the central nervous system (CNS). CBr2 is mainly expressed in the immune system and peripheral tissues. Additionally CBr1 and CBr2 are also present in keratinocytes [2]. Several studies provide evidence that cannabinoids may be effective in treatment of cancer pain and/or inhibition of tumor growth in cancers such as glioma, bone and skin squamous cell carcinoma [2,4,15,25,27].

For many years cannabinoids have been used for medicinal and recreational purposes. Recently, studies have focused on the therapeutic effects of cannabinoids on different cancers. The current study was the first to investigate the therapeutic effects of synthetic cannabinoids on oral cancer. Our results suggest that systemic administration of cannabinoids decease oral cancer pain. We have previously demonstrated the effects of morphine, which is the first line of treatment for pain in cancer patients, on paw withdrawal using the cancer pain mouse model [28]. Morphine reversed cancer-induced reductions in paw withdrawal threshold by 40–50%. In comparison, cannabinoid receptor agonists reversed cancer-induced pain (40% of control) with similar efficacy without the sedating/tolerance side effects of opioids. The present findings suggest that cannabinoid treatment may be a promising alternative therapy for oral cancer pain management. Furthermore, CBr2 agonism is not only palliative, but it may also be effective in inhibiting oral cancer growth, making the agonist a particularly desirable therapeutic agent."

Complete Study Links:

https://www.ncbi.nlm.nih.gov/pmc/articles/PMC3099480/
https://www.ncbi.nlm.nih.gov/pmc/articles/PMC3099480/pdf/nihms26088
6.pdf

The expression level of CB1 and CB2 receptors determines their efficacy at inducing apoptosis in astrocytomas.

PLoS One.

Eiron Cudaback,[1] William Marrs,[1,2] Thomas Moeller,[3] and Nephi Stella[1,4,*]

Joseph Najbauer, Editor

[1]Department of Pharmacology, University of Washington, Seattle, Washington, United States of America

[2] Graduate Program in Neurobiology and Behavior, University of Washington, Seattle, Washington, United States of America

[3] Department of Neurology, University of Washington, Seattle, Washington, United States of America

[4] Department of Psychiatry and Behavioral Sciences, University of Washington, Seattle, Washington, United States of America

City of Hope National Medical Center, United States of America

Abstract

BACKGROUND:

Cannabinoids represent unique compounds for treating tumors, including astrocytomas. Whether CB(1) and CB(2) receptors mediate this therapeutic effect is unclear.

PRINCIPAL FINDINGS:

We generated astrocytoma subclones that express set levels of CB(1) and CB(2), and found that cannabinoids induce apoptosis only in cells expressing low levels of receptors that couple to ERK1/2. In contrast, cannabinoids do not induce apoptosis in cells expressing high levels of receptors because these now also couple to the prosurvival signal AKT. Remarkably, cannabinoids applied at high concentration induce apoptosis in all subclones independently of CB(1), CB(2) and AKT, but still through a mechanism involving ERK1/2.

SIGNIFICANCE:

The high expression level of CB(1) and CB(2) receptors commonly found in malignant astrocytomas precludes the use of cannabinoids as therapeutics, unless AKT is concomitantly inhibited, or cannabinoids are applied at concentrations that bypass CB(1) and CB(2) receptors, yet still activate ERK1/2.

PubMed Link: http://www.ncbi.nlm.nih.gov/pubmed/20090845

Full Text: https://www.ncbi.nlm.nih.gov/pmc/articles/PMC2806825/

Cannabinoid receptors, CB1 and CB2, as novel targets for inhibition of non-small cell lung cancer growth and metastasis.

Cancer Prevention Research (Phila).
Preet A, Qamri Z, Nasser MW, Prasad A, Shilo K,
Zou X, Groopman JE, Ganju RK.
Division of Experimental Medicine, Beth Israel Deaconess Medical Center, Harvard Medical School, Boston, Massachusetts, USA.

Abstract

Non-small cell lung cancer (NSCLC) is the leading cause of cancer deaths worldwide; however, only limited therapeutic treatments are available. Hence, we investigated the role of cannabinoid receptors, CB1 and CB2, as novel therapeutic targets against NSCLC. We observed expression of CB1 (24%) and CB2 (55%) in NSCLC patients. Furthermore, we have shown that the treatment of NSCLC cell lines (A549 and SW-1573) with CB1/CB2- and CB2-specific agonists Win55,212-2 and JWH-015, respectively, significantly attenuated random as well as growth factor-directed in vitro chemotaxis and chemoinvasion in these cells. We also observed significant reduction in focal adhesion complex, which plays an important role in migration, upon treatment with both JWH-015 and Win55,212-2. In addition, pretreatment with CB1/CB2 selective antagonists, AM251 and AM630, prior to JWH-015 and Win55,212-2 treatments, attenuated the agonist-mediated inhibition of in vitro chemotaxis and chemoinvasion. In addition, both CB1 and CB2 agonists Win55,212-2 and JWH-133, respectively, significantly inhibited in vivo tumor growth and lung metastasis ($\sim$ 50%). These effects were receptor mediated, as pretreatment with CB1/CB2 antagonists abrogated CB1/CB2 agonist-mediated effects on tumor growth and metastasis. Reduced proliferation and vascularization, along with increased apoptosis, were observed in tumors obtained from animals treated with JWH-133 and Win55,212-2. Upon further elucidation into the molecular mechanism, we observed that both CB1 and CB2 agonists inhibited phosphorylation of AKT, a key signaling molecule controlling cell survival, migration, and apoptosis, and reduced matrix metalloproteinase 9 expression and activity. These results suggest that CB1 and CB2 could be used as novel therapeutic targets against NSCLC.

PubMed Link: https://www.ncbi.nlm.nih.gov/pubmed/21097714

FROM FULL TEXT:

"Non-small cell lung cancer (NSCLC), particularly metastatic lung cancer which accounts for approximately 85% of lung cancer cases, and is the leading cause of cancer-related mortality in the United States (1). Fewer than 15% of patients survive beyond 5 years after diagnosis....Consequently, there is a need for alternate therapy where other receptors specifically expressed on tumor cells can be targeted to abrogate EGFR-mediated signaling events directly or indirectly. In the present study, therefore, we analyzed the role of cannabinoid receptors CB1 and CB2 in NSCLC growth and metastasis.

There are three general types of cannabinoids: phytocannabinoids, THC and car-binodiol, are derived from plants; endogenous cannabinoids, 2AG and AEA, which are produced inside the body; and synthetic cannabinoids, JWH-133/JWH-015, CP-55 and Win55,212-2. These cannabinoids bind to two different cell surface G-protein coupled receptors, CB1 and CB2. CB1 receptor is predominantly expressed in the central nervous system (8,9), whereas CB2 receptor is expressed by immune cells (10). Recently, CB1 and CB2 have been shown to be overexpressed on tumor cells compared to normal cells in various types of cancers, such as breast (11) and liver (12), and therefore could be used as novel targets for cancer....The use of cannabinoid related drugs for medicinal purposes can be limited due to concerns of their psychotropic effects. We show for the first time that CB1 and CB2 receptors are overexpressed in NSCLC lung patient tissue samples. Furthermore, non-psychoactive small molecular weight synthetic cannabinoids inhibited growth, migration and invasion of NSCLC cells in in vitro as well as in vivo in a mouse model. In addition, molecular mechanism of inhibition reveals synthetic cannabinoid agonists may inhibit tumor growth and metastasis by inhibiting AKT phosphorylation and formation of focal adhesion structures. Our results suggest the use of non-psychoactive synthetic cannabinoid ligands as a promising strategy for inhibiting growth and metastasis of highly resistant NSCLC. Overall, our results indicate a novel role for cannabinoid receptors CB1 and CB2 in NSCLC growth and metastasis."

Complete Study Links:

http://cancerpreventionresearch.aacrjournals.org/content/4/1/65.long
https://www.ncbi.nlm.nih.gov/pmc/articles/PMC3025486/
https://www.ncbi.nlm.nih.gov/pmc/articles/PMC3025486/pdf/nihms25429
5.pdf

Cannabinoid CB1 receptor is downregulated in clear cell renal cell carcinoma.

Journal of Histochemistry and Cytochemistry.

Larrinaga G, Sanz B, Pérez I, Blanco L, Cándenas ML, Pinto FM, Gil J, López JI.Author information
Department of Physiology, Faculty of Medicine and Dentistry, University of the Basque Country, Universidad del País Vasco/Euskal Herriko Unibertsitatea (UPV/EHU), Leioa, Bizkaia, Spain.

Abstract
Several studies in cell cultures and in animal models have demonstrated that cannabinoids have important antitumoral properties. Because many of these effects are mediated through cannabinoid (CB) receptors CB1 and CB2, the study of their expression in human neoplasms has become of great interest in recent years. Fresh and formalin-fixed tissue samples of 20 consecutive clear cell renal cell carcinomas (CCRCCs) were collected prospectively and analyzed for the expression of both CB receptors by using RT-PCR,

Western blot (WB), and immunohistochemical techniques. RT-PCR assays demonstrated the expression of mRNA encoding the CB₁ in tumor tissue and in adjacent non-neoplastic kidney. Conversely, WB and IHC revealed a marked downregulation of CB1 protein in tumor tissue; CB1 was not expressed. The obtained data suggest a possible implication of the endocannabinoid system in renal carcinogenesis. A posttranscriptional downregulation of CB1 and the absence of expression of CB2 characterize CCRCC.

PubMed Link: https://www.ncbi.nlm.nih.gov/pubmed/20852034

FROM FULL TEXT:

"In the last decade, several studies in cell cultures and in animal models have demonstrated that CBs have proapoptotic, antiproliferative, antimetastatic, and antiangiogenic effects in various cancer types (Alexander et al. 2009). Although no clinical basis exists to recommend the use of natural/synthetic CBs in patients with renal cancer, this knowledge has spurred a clinical trial examining the efficacy and safety of giving D9- tetrahydrocannabinol locally to patients with other neoplasias, such as recurrent glioblastoma multiforme (Guzmán et al. 2006). Because many of these antitumoral effects of cannabinoids are mediated through CB receptors, the analysis of the expression of CB1 and CB2 receptors in a wide variety of human neoplasms has become of great interest, with some promising results appearing in the recent literature (Flygare and Sander 2008; Alpini and DeMorrow 2009). Although CCRCC is a paradigm of multi–antitumoral-drug-resistant neoplasia, a study on the role of ECS on this tumor is lacking

The precise role of the CB1 in renal cancer still remains to be clarified. It should be noted that a similar CB receptor expression profile has been reported recently in human colorectal cancer by Wang et al. (2008). The authors have suggested that CB1 loss would make cancer cells resistant to the antitumoral effect of endo-cannabinoids, thus accelerating intestinal tumor growth and biological aggres-siveness (Wang et al. 2008). This evidence favors the hypothesis that CB1 downregulation is a general mechanism in some different cancer types. In this sense, Caffarel et al. (2006) also observed downregulation of CB1 in human breast cancer cells. However, CB1 upregulation has also been reported in other human neoplasms, such as prostatic adenocarcinoma (Sarfaraz et al. 2005), hepa-tocellular carcinoma (Xu et al. 2006), and pancreatic ductal adenocarcinoma (Carracedo et al. 2006; Michalski et al. 2008). Therefore, further studies are needed to clarify the precise mechanisms underlying these apparently divergent results."

Complete Study Links:
https://www.ncbi.nlm.nih.gov/pmc/articles/PMC2989249/
https://www.ncbi.nlm.nih.gov/pmc/articles/PMC2989249/pdf/1129.pdf

A combined preclinical therapy of cannabinoids and temozolomide against glioma.

Molecular Cancer Theraputics.

Torres S, Lorente M, Rodríguez-Fornés F, Hernández-Tiedra S, Salazar M, García-Taboada E, Barcia J, Guzmán M, Velasco G.
Department of Biochemistry and Molecular Biology I, School of Biology, Complutense University, C/José Antonio Novais, Madrid, Spain.

Abstract

Glioblastoma multiforme (GBM) is highly resistant to current anticancer treatments, which makes it crucial to find new therapeutic strategies aimed at improving the poor prognosis of patients suffering from this disease. $\Delta(9)$-Tetrahydrocannabinol (THC), the major active ingredient of marijuana, and other cannabinoid receptor agonists inhibit tumor growth in animal models of cancer, including glioma, an effect that relies, at least in part, on the stimulation of autophagy-mediated apoptosis in tumor cells. Here, we show that the combined administration of THC and temozolomide (TMZ; the benchmark agent for the management of GBM) exerts a strong antitumoral action in glioma xenografts, an effect that is also observed in tumors that are resistant to TMZ treatment. Combined administration of THC and TMZ enhanced autophagy, whereas pharmacologic or genetic inhibition of this process prevented TMZ + THC-induced cell death, supporting that activation of autophagy plays a crucial role on the mechanism of action of this drug combination. Administration of submaximal doses of THC and cannabidiol (CBD; another plant-derived cannabinoid that also induces glioma cell death through a mechanism of action different from that of THC) remarkably reduces the growth of glioma xenografts. Moreover, treatment with TMZ and submaximal doses of THC and CBD produced a strong antitumoral action in both TMZ-sensitive and TMZ-resistant tumors. Altogether, our findings support that the combined administration of TMZ and cannabinoids could be therapeutically exploited for the management of GBM.

PubMed Link: https://www.ncbi.nlm.nih.gov/pubmed/21220494

FROM FULL TEXT:

"Combined treatment with THC and TMZ strongly reduces the growth of glioma xenografts To analyze the combined antitumoral action ofTMZ and THC in gliomas, we first characterized the ability of the 2 individual agents to promote glioma cell death. In agreement with the results obtained by other groups (29, 30), we observed that TMZ treatment produced a dose-dependent reduction incell viability that reached a value of 40%to 50% of viable cells even when high concentrations of this agent (up to 400 mmol/L) were used (Supplementary Fig. 2A). Likewise, THC reduced in a dose-dependent manner the viability of glioma cells (Supplementary Fig. 2B).Wetherefore selected submaximal doses of TMZ and THC to evaluate whether the combined administration of the 2 agents enhanced their ability to induce glioma celldeath. In line with this possibility, combined treatment with low doses of THC and TMZ reduced in a synergic fashion the viability of several human glioma cell lines and of 2 primary cultures of glioma cells derived from human GBM biopsies (Fig. 1A andSupplementary Fig. 2B).

160

Cannabinoids, a new family of potential anticancer compounds, are devoid of the strong side effects associated with other chemotherapeutic agents (10, 46). Thus, no signs of toxicity were observed in patients enrolled in a pilot clinical trial for the treatment of GBM with THC (17) or in tumor-bearing animals treated intracranially, peritumorally, or intraperitoneally with THC (refs. 14, 18; data not shown). Moreover, no overt toxic effects have been reported in other clinical trials with cannabinoids (including Sativex) in cancer patients for various applications (e.g., inhibition of nausea, vomiting, and pain), using different routes of administration (e.g., oral, oromucosal; refs. 11, 47). These characteristics, together with their remarkable anticancer activity, make cannabinoids excellent candidate drugs for combination with other antineoplastic agents. Results presented here specifically show that the coadministration of TMZ with THC and with-THCþ CBD exerts a strong antitumoral action in glioma xenografts."

Complete Study Links:

http://mct.aacrjournals.org/content/10/1/90.long
http://mct.aacrjournals.org/content/molcanther/10/1/90.full.pdf

Update on the endocannabinoid system as an anticancer target.

Expert Opinion on Theraputic Targets.
Malfitano AM, Ciaglia E, Gangemi G,
Gazzerro P, Laezza C, Bifulco M.
University of Salerno, Department of Pharmaceutical Sciences, Fisciano, Salerno, Italy.

Abstract
INTRODUCTION:
Recent studies have shown that the endocannabinoid system (ECS) could offer an attractive antitumor target. Numerous findings suggest the involvement of this system (constituted mainly by cannabinoid receptors, endogenous compounds and the enzymes for their synthesis and degradation) in cancer cell growth in vitro and in vivo.
AREAS COVERED:
This review covers literature from the past decade which highlights the potential of targeting the ECS for cancer treatment. In particular, the levels of endocannabinoids and the expression of their receptors in several types of cancer are discussed, along with the signaling pathways involved in the endocannabinoid antitumor effects. Furthermore, the beneficial and adverse effects of old and novel compounds in clinical use are discussed.
EXPERT OPINION:
One direction that should be pursued in antitumor therapy is to select compounds with reduced psychoactivity. This is known to be connected to the CB1 receptor; thus, targeting the CB2 receptor is a popular objective. CB1 receptors could be maintained as a target to design new compounds, and mixed CB1-CB2 ligands could be effective if they are able to not cross the BBB. Furthermore, targeting the ECS with agents that activate cannabinoid receptors or inhibitors of endogenous degrading systems such as fatty acid amide hydrolase inhibitors may have relevant therapeutic impact on tumor growth. Additional studies into

the downstream consequences of endocannabinoid treatment are required and may illuminate other potential therapeutic targets.

PubMed Link: https://www.ncbi.nlm.nih.gov/pubmed/21244344

Cannabinoids, Endocannabinoids and Cancer
Cancer Metastasis

Daniel J. Hermanson and Lawrence J. Marnett
A.B Hancock Jr. Memorial Laboratory for Cancer Research, Departments of Biochemistry,
Chemistry, and Pharmacology, Vanderbilt Institute of Chemical Biology, Center in Molecular
Toxicology, Vanderbilt Ingram Comprehensive Cancer Center, Vanderbilt University School of
Medicine, Nashville TN

Abstract
Many laboratories have proposed that cannabinoids and endocannabinoids directly inhibit tumor growth in vitro and in animal tumor models through several different pathways. The inhibition of tumor growth and progression of several types of cancers including glioma, glioblastoma, breast cancer, prostate cancer, thyroid cancer, colon carcinoma, leukemia, and lymphoid tumors have been demonstrated by natural and synthetic cannabinoids, endocannabinoids, endocannabinoid analogs, endocannabinoid transport inhibitors, and endocannabinoid degradation inhibitors.

PubMed Link:
https://www.ncbi.nlm.nih.gov/pmc/articles/PMC3366283/pdf/nihms-373922.pdf

Crosstalk between chemokine receptor CXCR4 and cannabinoid receptor CB2 in modulating breast cancer growth and invasion.
PLoS One.

Nasser MW, Qamri Z, Deol YS, Smith D, Shilo K, Zou X, Ganju RK.
Department of Pathology and Comprehensive Cancer Center, The Ohio State University, Columbus, Ohio, United States of America.

Abstract
BACKGROUND:
Cannabinoids bind to cannabinoid receptors CB(1) and CB(2) and have been reported to possess anti-tumorigenic activity in various cancers. However, the mechanisms through which cannabinoids modulate tumor growth are not well known. In this study, we report that a synthetic non-psychoactive cannabinoid that specifically binds to cannabinoid receptor CB(2) may modulate breast tumor growth and metastasis by inhibiting signaling

of the chemokine receptor CXCR4 and its ligand CXCL12. This signaling pathway has been shown to play an important role in regulating breast cancer progression and metastasis.

METHODOLOGY/PRINCIPAL FINDINGS:

We observed high expression of both CB(2) and CXCR4 receptors in breast cancer patient tissues by immunohistochemical analysis. We further found that CB(2)-specific agonist JWH-015 inhibits the CXCL12-induced chemotaxis and wound healing of MCF7 overexpressing CXCR4 (MCF7/CXCR4), highly metastatic clone of MDA-MB-231 (SCP2) and NT 2.5 cells (derived from MMTV-neu) by using chemotactic and wound healing assays. Elucidation of the molecular mechanisms using various biochemical techniques and confocal microscopy revealed that JWH-015 treatment inhibited CXCL12-induced P44/P42 ERK activation, cytoskeletal focal adhesion and stress fiber formation, which play a critical role in breast cancer invasion and metastasis. In addition, we have shown that JWH-015 significantly inhibits orthotopic tumor growth in syngenic mice in vivo using NT 2.5 cells. Furthermore, our studies have revealed that JWH-015 significantly inhibits phosphorylation of CXCR4 and its downstream signaling in vivo in orthotopic and spontaneous breast cancer MMTV-PyMT mouse model systems.

CONCLUSIONS/SIGNIFICANCE:

This study provides novel insights into the crosstalk between CB(2) and CXCR4/CXCL12-signaling pathways in the modulation of breast tumor growth and metastasis. Furthermore, these studies indicate that CB(2) receptors could be used for developing innovative therapeutic strategies against breast cancer.

PubMed Link: https://www.ncbi.nlm.nih.gov/pubmed/21915267

FROM FULL TEXT:

"Breast cancer is the second leading cause of cancer death in women in the United States. Despite recent advances in hormonal therapies, mortality still remains high due to breast cancer metastasis to other organs. Synthetic cannabinoids that bind to cannabinoid receptors CB1 and CB2 have been shown to inhibit migration, metastasis, and invasion of various cell types including breast cancer cells [4,5,6,37,41] The results of this study suggest that CB2-specific nonpsychoactive synthetic cannabinoid JWH-015 inhibits CXCL12-induced migration and invasive properties of breast cancer cells. Furthermore, elucidation of signaling mechanisms reveals that JWH-015 inhibits CXCL12-induced CXCR4 and ERK phosphorylation, focal adhesion formation and actin stress fiber polymerization. Thus, we conclude that CB2-specific synthetic cannabinoids that do not possess psychoactivity can be developed to design novel therapies against breast cancer growth and metastasis by blocking CXCR4/CXCL12-induced signaling."

Complete Study Links:

https://www.ncbi.nlm.nih.gov/pmc/articles/PMC3168464/
https://www.ncbi.nlm.nih.gov/pmc/articles/PMC3168464/pdf/pone.00239 01.pdf

Antiproliferative mechanism of a cannabinoid agonist by cell cycle arrest in human gastric cancer cells.

Journal of Cellular Biochemistry.

Park JM, Xian XS, Choi MG, Park H, Cho YK, Lee IS, Kim SW, Chung IS.
Division of Gastroenterology, Department of Internal Medicine, College of Medicine, The Catholic University of Korea, Seoul, Korea.

Abstract (edited):

"For gastric cancers, the antineoplastic activity of cannabinoids has been investigated in only a few reports and knowledge regarding the mechanisms involved is limited. We have reported previously that treatment of gastric cancer cells with a cannabinoid agonist significantly decreased cell proliferation and induced apoptosis. Here, we evaluated the effects of cannabinoids on various cellular mediators involved in cell cycle arrest in gastric cancer cells. AGS and MKN-1 cell lines were used as human gastric cancer cells and WIN 55,212-2 as a cannabinoid agonist....Cell cycle arrest preceded apoptotic response. Thus, this cannabinoid agonist can reduce gastric cancer cell proliferation via G1 phase cell cycle arrest, which is mediated via activation of the MAPK pathway and inhibition of pAKT."

PubMed Link: https://www.ncbi.nlm.nih.gov/pubmed/21312237

note: the following is a case study of two children with tumors that regressed after smoking marijuana

Spontaneous regression of septum pellucidum/forniceal pilocytic astrocytomas--possible role of Cannabis inhalation.

International Society for Pediactric Neurosurgery

Foroughi M, Hendson G, Sargent MA, Steinbok P.
Division of Pediatric Neurosurgery, Department of Surgery, BC Children's Hospital, Vancouver, BC, Canada.

Abstract

INTRODUCTION:
Spontaneous regression of pilocytic astrocytoma after incomplete resection is well recognized, especially for cerebellar and optic pathway tumors, and tumors associated with Neurofibromatosis type-1 (NF1). The purpose of this report is to document spontaneous regression of pilocytic astrocytomas of the septum pellucidum and to discuss the possible role of cannabis in promoting regression.
CASE REPORT:
We report two children with septum pellucidum/forniceal pilocytic astrocytoma (PA) tumors in the absence of NF-1, who underwent craniotomy and subtotal excision, leaving behind a small residual in each case. During Magnetic Resonance Imaging (MRI) surveillance in the first three years, one case was dormant and the other showed slight increase in size, followed by clear regression of both residual tumors over the following 3-year period. Neither patient received any conventional adjuvant treatment. The tumors regressed over

the same period of time that cannabis was consumed via inhalation, raising the possibility that the cannabis played a role in the tumor regression.

CONCLUSION:

We advise caution against instituting adjuvant therapy or further aggressive surgery for small residual PAs, especially in eloquent locations, even if there appears to be slight progression, since regression may occur later. Further research may be appropriate to elucidate the increasingly recognized effect of cannabis/cannabinoids on gliomas.

PubMed Link: https://www.ncbi.nlm.nih.gov/pubmed/21336992

Gemcitabine/cannabinoid combination triggers autophagy in pancreatic cancer cells through a ROS-mediated mechanism.

Cell Death and Disease.

Donadelli M, Dando I, Zaniboni T, Costanzo C, Dalla Pozza E, Scupoli MT, Scarpa A, Zappavigna S, Marra M, Abbruzzese A, Bifulco M, Caraglia M, Palmieri M.

Department of Life and Reproduction Sciences, Biochemistry Section, University of Verona, Verona, Italy.

Abstract

Gemcitabine (GEM, 2',2'-difluorodeoxycytidine) is currently used in advanced pancreatic adenocarcinoma, with a response rate of < 20%. The purpose of our work was to improve GEM activity by addition of cannabinoids. Here, we show that GEM induces both cannabinoid receptor-1 (CB1) and cannabinoid receptor-2 (CB2) receptors by an NF-κB-dependent mechanism and that its association with cannabinoids synergistically inhibits pancreatic adenocarcinoma cell growth and increases reactive oxygen species (ROS) induced by single treatments. The antiproliferative synergism is prevented by the radical scavenger N-acetyl-L-cysteine and by the specific NF-κB inhibitor BAY 11-7085, demonstrating that the induction of ROS by GEM/cannabinoids and of NF-κB by GEM is required for this effect. In addition, we report that neither apoptotic nor cytostatic mechanisms are responsible for the synergistic cell growth inhibition, which is strictly associated with the enhancement of endoplasmic reticulum stress and autophagic cell death. Noteworthy, the antiproliferative synergism is stronger in GEM-resistant pancreatic cancer cell lines compared with GEM-sensitive pancreatic cancer cell lines. The combined treatment strongly inhibits growth of human pancreatic tumor cells xenografted in nude mice without apparent toxic effects. These findings support a key role of the ROS-dependent activation of an autophagic program in the synergistic growth inhibition induced by GEM/cannabinoid combination in human pancreatic cancer cells.

PubMed Link: https://www.ncbi.nlm.nih.gov/pubmed/21525939

FROM FULL TEXT:

"In the present study, we have demonstrated that the combination between the standard chemotherapy agent GEM and cannabinoids synergistically inhibited pancreatic adenocarcinoma cell growth by a ROS-dependent autophagic cell death. We used highly specific cannabinoid ligands of CB1 (ACPA) and CB2 (GW), and the clinically relevant CB1 ligand SR1. The latter has been described as a CB1 antagonist or inverse agonist;23 however, at high concentration it possesses an agonist activity. Our results were in agreement with the last observation and additionally confirmed the dual and concentration-dependent effect of SR1 on cell response (data not shown). SR1 counteracts obesity and its metabolic complications regulating food intake at central and peripheral level25 and also exerts antitumoral activity in some cancer types and in thyroid tumor xenografts. In contrast to SR1, to our knowledge, the antitumor activity of ACPA and GW has never been reported before. Thus, our results show for the first time that GW, ACPA, or SR1, in addition to GEM, were able to synergistically inhibit pancreatic adenocarcinoma cell growth."

Complete Study Links:
https://www.ncbi.nlm.nih.gov/pmc/articles/PMC3122066/
https://www.ncbi.nlm.nih.gov/pmc/articles/PMC3122066/pdf/cddis20113
6a.pdf

Cannabidiol induces programmed cell death in breast cancer cells by coordinating the cross-talk between apoptosis and autophagy.

Molecular Cancer Theraputics.
Shrivastava A, Kuzontkoski PM, Groopman JE, Prasad A.
Division of Experimental Medicine, Beth Israel Deaconess Medical Center, Boston, MA USA.

Abstract
Cannabidiol (CBD), a major nonpsychoactive constituent of cannabis, is considered an antineoplastic agent on the basis of its in vitro and in vivo activity against tumor cells. However, the exact molecular mechanism through which CBD mediates this activity is yet to be elucidated. Here, we have shown CBD-induced cell death of breast cancer cells, independent of cannabinoid and vallinoid receptor activation. Electron microscopy revealed morphologies consistent with the coexistence of autophagy and apoptosis. Western blot analysis confirmed these findings. We showed that CBD induces endoplasmic reticulum stress and, subsequently, inhibits AKT and mTOR signaling as shown by decreased levels of phosphorylated mTOR and 4EBP1, and cyclin D1. Analyzing further the cross-talk between the autophagic and apoptotic signaling pathways, we found that beclin1 plays a central role in the induction of CBD-mediated apoptosis in MDA-MB-231 breast cancer cells. Although CBD enhances the interaction between beclin1 and Vps34, it inhibits the association between beclin1 and Bcl-2. In addition, we showed that CBD reduces mitochondrial membrane potential, triggers the translocation of BID to the mitochondria, the release of cytochrome c to the cytosol, and, ultimately, the activation of the intrinsic apoptotic pathway in breast cancer cells. CBD increased the generation of reactive oxygen species (ROS), and ROS inhibition blocked the induction of apoptosis and autophagy. Our study revealed an intricate interplay between apoptosis and autophagy in CBD-treated

166

breast cancer cells and highlighted the value of continued investigation into the potential use of CBD as an antineoplastic agent.

PubMed Link: https://www.ncbi.nlm.nih.gov/pubmed/21566064

FROM FULL TEXT:

"There is an urgent need to develop innovative ways to treat breast cancer that has become resistant to established therapies. We sought to identify novel agents by examining natural products with validated, anticancer properties. We focused our study on the cannabinoid CBD, which induces cytotoxicity in human glioma, leukemia, and breast cancer cells in vitro (5, 8–12, 38) and inhibits the metastasis of breast cancer cells (12, 38). We explored the molecular mechanisms by which CBD induced PCD in breast cancer cells lines, and examined the intricate relationship between CBD-induced apoptosis, autophagy, and ROS generation. We found that CBD inhibited the survival of both estrogen receptor-positive and estrogen receptor-negative breast cancer cell lines and induced apoptosis in a concentration-dependent manner. Moreover, at these concentrations, CBD had little effect on MCF-10A cells, nontumorigenic, mammary cells (19). These data enhance the desirability of CBD as an anticancer agent, because they suggest that CBD preferentially kills breast cancer cells, while minimizing damage to normal breast tissue."

Complete Study Links:
http://mct.aacrjournals.org/content/10/7/1161.long
http://mct.aacrjournals.org/content/molcanther/10/7/1161.full.pdf

Anti-tumoral action of cannabinoids on hepatocellular carcinoma: role of AMPK-dependent activation of autophagy.

Cell Death and Diffentiation.
Vara D, Salazar M, Olea-Herrero N, Guzmán M,
Velasco G, Díaz-Laviada I.
Department of Biochemistry and Molecular Biology, School of Medicine,
Alcalá University, Madrid, Spain.

Abstract
Hepatocellular carcinoma (HCC) is the third cause of cancer-related death worldwide. When these tumors are in advanced stages, few therapeutic options are available. Therefore, it is essential to search for new treatments to fight this disease. In this study, we investigated the effects of cannabinoids--a novel family of potential anticancer agents--on the growth of HCC. We found that $\Delta(9)$-tetrahydrocannabinol ($\Delta(9)$-THC, the main active component of Cannabis sativa) and JWH-015 (a cannabinoid receptor 2 (CB(2)) cannabinoid receptor-selective agonist) reduced the viability of the human HCC cell lines HepG2 (human hepatocellular liver carcinoma cell line) and HuH-7 (hepatocellular carcinoma cells), an effect that relied on the stimulation of CB(2) receptor. We also found that

167

Δ(9)-THC- and JWH-015-induced autophagy relies on tribbles homolog 3 (TRB3) upregulation, and subsequent inhibition of the serine-threonine kinase Akt/mammalian target of rapamycin C1 axis and adenosine monophosphate-activated kinase (AMPK) stimulation. Pharmacological and genetic inhibition of AMPK upstream kinases supported that calmodulin-activated kinase kinase β was responsible for cannabinoid-induced AMPK activation and autophagy. In vivo studies revealed that Δ(9)-THC and JWH-015 reduced the growth of HCC subcutaneous xenografts, an effect that was not evident when autophagy was genetically of pharmacologically inhibited in those tumors. Moreover, cannabinoids were also able to inhibit tumor growth and ascites in an orthotopic model of HCC xenograft. Our findings may contribute to the design of new therapeutic strategies for the management of HCC.

PubMed Link: https://www.ncbi.nlm.nih.gov/pubmed/21475304

FROM FULL TEXT:
"This study was therefore undertaken to evaluate the potential anti-tumoral activity of cannabinoids in HCC and the mechanisms responsible for cannabinoid action in that devastating disease. We found that, both in cell cultures and in xenografted mice, D9-THC and the synthetic CB2 receptor-selective agonist JWH-015 promote human HCC death via autophagy stimulation. We also provide a molecular mechanism underlying CB2 receptor-mediated anti-tumoral signaling. These observations may pave the way to the design of novel therapeutic strategies for the treatment of hepatocellular carcinoma."

Complete Study Links:
https://www.ncbi.nlm.nih.gov/pmc/articles/PMC3131949/
https://www.ncbi.nlm.nih.gov/pmc/articles/PMC3131949/pdf/cdd201132a.pdf

Pathways mediating the effects of cannabidiol on the reduction of breast cancer cell proliferation, invasion, and metastasis.
Breast Cancer Research and Treatment.

McAllister SD, Murase R, Christian RT, Lau D, Zielinski AJ, Allison J, Almanza C, Pakdel A, Lee J, Limbad C, Liu Y, Debs RJ, Moore DH, Desprez PY.
California Pacific Medical Center, Research Institute, San Francisco, CA, USA.

Abstract
Invasion and metastasis of aggressive breast cancer cells are the final and fatal steps during cancer progression. Clinically, there are still limited therapeutic interventions for aggressive and metastatic breast cancers available. Therefore, effective, targeted, and non-toxic therapies are urgently required. Id-1, an inhibitor of basic helix-loop-helix transcription factors, has recently been shown to be a

key regulator of the metastatic potential of breast and additional cancers. We previously reported that cannabidiol (CBD), a cannabinoid with a low toxicity profile, down-regulated Id-1 gene expression in aggressive human breast cancer cells in culture. Using cell proliferation and invasion assays, cell flow cytometry to examine cell cycle and the formation of reactive oxygen species, and Western analysis, we determined pathways leading to the down-regulation of Id-1 expression by CBD and consequently to the inhibition of the proliferative and invasive phenotype of human breast cancer cells. Then, using the mouse 4T1 mammary tumor cell line and the ranksum test, two different syngeneic models of tumor metastasis to the lungs were chosen to determine whether treatment with CBD would reduce metastasis in vivo. We show that CBD inhibits human breast cancer cell proliferation and invasion through differential modulation of the extracellular signal-regulated kinase (ERK) and reactive oxygen species (ROS) pathways, and that both pathways lead to down-regulation of Id-1 expression. Moreover, we demonstrate that CBD up-regulates the pro-differentiation factor, Id-2. Using immune competent mice, we then show that treatment with CBD significantly reduces primary tumor mass as well as the size and number of lung metastatic foci in two models of metastasis. Our data demonstrate the efficacy of CBD in pre-clinical models of breast cancer. The results have the potential to lead to the development of novel non-toxic compounds for the treatment of breast cancer metastasis, and the information gained from these experiments broaden our knowledge of both Id-1 and cannabinoid biology as it pertains to cancer progression.

PubMed Link: https://www.ncbi.nlm.nih.gov/pubmed/20859676

FROM FULL TEXT:

"The path of cancer progression is determined by alterations in the regulatory mechanisms of growth/invasion and differentiation. The expression of Id-1 protein (an inhibitor of basic helix-loop-helix transcription factors) has been reported to be dysregulated in over 20 types of cancer, and suggested as a key determinant of tumorigenesis and/or metastasis in a wide range of tissues, including the breast [34, 35]. Reducing Id-1 expression (a gene whose expression is absent in most of the healthy adult tissues) could therefore provide a rational therapeutic strategy for the treatment of aggressive cancers. Our previous data suggested that CBD represented a non-toxic plant derived compound that could reduce Id-1 expression and corresponding breast cancer metastasis [21]. A key piece of data that was needed in order to increase enthusiasm for the development of future clinical trials was the establishment of molecular pathways leading to reduction of Id-1 expression and corresponding breast cancer metastasis."

Complete Study Links:

https://www.ncbi.nlm.nih.gov/pmc/articles/PMC3410650/
https://www.ncbi.nlm.nih.gov/pmc/articles/PMC3410650/pdf/nihms39507
0.pdf

The endocannabinoid system and cancer: therapeutic implication.

British Journal of Pharmacology

Guindon J, Hohmann AG.
Department of Psychological and Brain Sciences, Indiana University, Bloomington, IN , USA.

Abstract (edited):
"The endocannabinoid system is implicated in a variety of physiological and pathological conditions (inflammation, immunomodulation, analgesia, cancer and others). The main active ingredient of cannabis, $\Delta(9)$ -tetrahydrocannabinol ($\Delta(9)$ -THC), produces its effects through activation of CB(1) and CB(2) receptors.... cannabis-like compounds offer therapeutic potential for the treatment of breast, prostate and bone cancer in patients. Further basic research on anti-cancer properties of cannabinoids as well as clinical trials of cannabinoid therapeutic efficacy in breast, prostate and bone cancer is therefore warranted."

PubMed Link: https://www.ncbi.nlm.nih.gov/pubmed/21410463

Complete Study Links:
https://www.ncbi.nlm.nih.gov/pmc/articles/PMC3165955/
https://www.ncbi.nlm.nih.gov/pmc/articles/PMC3165955/pdf/bph0163-1447.pdf

2012

Cannabinoid-associated cell death mechanisms in tumor models (review).

International Journal of Oncology

Calvaruso G, Pellerito O, Notaro A, Giuliano M.
Department of Experimental Biomedicine and Clinical Neuroscience, University of Palermo, Palermo, Italy.

Abstract
In recent years, cannabinoids (the active components of Cannabis sativa) and their derivatives have received considerable interest due to findings that they can affect the viability and invasiveness of a variety of different cancer cells. Moreover, in addition to their inhibitory effects on tumor growth and migration, angiogenesis and metastasis, the ability of these compounds to induce different pathways of cell death has been highlighted. Here, we review the most recent results generating interest in the field of death mechanisms induced by cannabinoids in cancer cells. In particular, we analyze the pathways triggered by cannabinoids to induce apoptosis or autophagy and investigate the interplay between the two processes. Overall, the results reported here suggest that the

exploration of molecular mechanisms induced by cannabinoids in cancer cells can contribute to the development of safe and effective treatments in cancer therapy.

PubMed Link: https://www.ncbi.nlm.nih.gov/pubmed/22614735

Cannabinoids: a new hope for breast cancer therapy?
Cancer Treat Reviews

Caffarel MM, Andradas C, Pérez-Gómez E, Guzmán M, Sánchez C.
Dept. Biochemistry and Molecular Biology I, School of Biology, Complutense University-CIBERNED-IRYCIS, Madrid, Spain.

Abstract (edited):
"Experimental evidence accumulated during the last decade supports that cannabinoids, the active components of Cannabis sativa and their derivatives, possess anticancer activity. Thus, these compounds exert anti-proliferative, pro-apoptotic, anti-migratory and anti-invasive actions in a wide spectrum of cancer cells in culture. Moreover, tumor growth, angiogenesis and metastasis are hampered by cannabinoids in xenograft-based and genetically-engineered mouse models of cancer. This review summarizes our current knowledge on the anti-tumor potential of cannabinoids in breast cancer, which suggests that cannabinoid-based medicines may be useful for the treatment of most breast tumor subtypes."

PubMed Link: https://www.ncbi.nlm.nih.gov/pubmed/22776349

Cannabidiolic acid, a major cannabinoid in fiber-type cannabis, is an inhibitor of MDA-MB-231 breast cancer cell migration.
Toxicology Letters

Takeda S, Okajima S, Miyoshi H, Yoshida K, Okamoto Y, Okada T, Amamoto T, Watanabe K, Omiecinski CJ, Aramaki H.
Department of Molecular Biology, Daiichi University of Pharmacy, Tamagawa-cho, Minami-ku, Fukuoka, Japan.

Abstract (edited):
"Cannabidiol (CBD), a major non-psychotropic constituent of fiber-type cannabis plant, has been reported to possess diverse biological activities, including anti-proliferative effect on cancer cells...Results of the current investigation revealed that CBDA inhibits migration of the highly invasive MDA-MB-231 human breast cancer cells, apparently through a mechanism involving inhibition of cAMP-dependent protein kinase...The data presented in this report suggest for the first time that as an active component in the cannabis plant, CBDA offers potential therapeutic modality in the abrogation of cancer cell migration, including aggressive breast cancers.

PubMed Link: https://www.ncbi.nlm.nih.gov/pubmed/22963825

Non-THC cannabinoids inhibit prostate carcinoma growth in vitro and in vivo: pro-apoptotic effects and underlying mechanisms.

British Journal of Pharmacology.

De Petrocellis L, Ligresti A, Schiano Moriello A, Iappelli M, Verde R, Stott CG, Cristino L, Orlando P, Di Marzo V.

Istituto di Cibernetica, Endocannabinoid Research Group, Consiglio Nazionale delle Ricerche, Pozzuoli, Italy.

Abstract (edited):

"Cannabinoid receptor activation induces prostate carcinoma cell (PCC) apoptosis, but cannabinoids other than Δ(9) -tetrahydrocannabinol (THC), which lack potency at cannabinoid receptors, have not been investigated...We tested pure cannabinoids and extracts from Cannabis strains enriched in particular cannabinoids (BDS), on AR-positive (LNCaP and 22RV1) and -negative (DU-145 and PC-3) cells, by evaluating cell viability (MTT test), cell cycle arrest and apoptosis induction, by FACS scans, caspase 3/7 assays, DNA fragmentation and TUNEL, and size of xenograft tumours induced by LNCaP and DU-145 cells....Cannabidiol (CBD) significantly inhibited cell viability. Other compounds became effective in cells deprived of serum for 24 h."

PubMed Link: https://www.ncbi.nlm.nih.gov/pubmed/22594963

Critical appraisal of the potential use of cannabinoids in cancer management.

Cancer Management Research

Cridge BJ, Rosengren RJ.

Department of Pharmacology and Toxicology, University of Otago, Dunedin, New Zealand.

Abstract:

Cannabinoids have been attracting a great deal of interest as potential anticancer agents. Originally derived from the plant Cannabis sativa, there are now a number of endo-, phyto- and synthetic cannabinoids available. This review summarizes the key literature to date around the actions, antitumor activity, and mechanisms of action for this broad range of compounds. Cannabinoids are largely defined by an ability to activate the cannabinoid receptors - CB1 or CB2. The action of the cannabinoids is very dependent on the exact ligand tested, the dose, and the duration of exposure. Some cannabinoids, synthetic or plant-derived, show potential as therapeutic agents, and evidence across a range of cancers and evidence in vitro and in vivo is starting to be accumulated. Studies have now been conducted in a wide range of cell lines, including glioma, breast, prostate, endothelial, liver, and lung. This work is complemented by an increasing body of evidence from in vivo models. However, many of these results remain contradictory, an issue that is not currently able to be resolved through current knowledge of mechanisms of action. While there is a developing understanding of potential mechanisms of action, with the extracellular signal-regulated kinase pathway emerging as a critical signaling juncture in combination with an important role for ceramide and lipid signaling, the relative importance of each pathway is yet to be determined. The interplay between the intracellular pathways of autophagy versus apoptosis is a recent development that is discussed. Overall, there is still a great deal of conflicting evidence around the future utility of the cannabinoids, natural or synthetic, as therapeutic agents.

PubMed Link: https://www.ncbi.nlm.nih.gov/pubmed/24039449

Towards the use of non-psychoactive cannabinoids for prostate cancer.

British Journal of Pharmacology
Pacher P.
Section on Oxidative Stress Tissue Injury, Laboratory of Physiological Studies, National Institutes of Health, NIAAA, Bethesda, MD, USA.

Abstract:
The palliative effects of Cannabis sativa (marijuana), and its putative main active ingredient, $\Delta(9)$ -tetrahydrocannabinol (THC), which include appetite stimulation, attenuation of nausea and emesis associated with chemo- or radiotherapy, pain relief, mood elevation, and relief from insomnia in cancer patients, are well-known. Because of the adverse psychoactive effects of THC, numerous recent preclinical studies have been focused on investigating other non-psychoactive constituents of C. sativa, such as cannabidiol, for potential therapeutic use. In this issue of the British Journal of Pharmacology, De Petrocellis and colleagues present comprehensive evidence that plant-derived cannabinoids, especially cannabidiol, are potent inhibitors of prostate carcinoma viability in vitro. They also showed that the extract was active in vivo, either alone or when administered with drugs commonly used to treat prostate cancer (the anti-mitotic chemotherapeutic drug docetaxel (Taxotere) or the anti-androgen bicalutamide (Casodex)) and explored the potential mechanisms behind these antineoplastic effects.

PubMed Link: https://www.ncbi.nlm.nih.gov/pmc/articles/PMC3570005/

Cannabis Oil was given to this patient late in her illness, after all conventional therapies were used. Although this patient died, the blood work revealed the cancer in the white blood cells decreased, according to the administration of Cannabis Oil.

Cannabis extract treatment for terminal acute lymphoblastic leukemia with a Philadelphia chromosome mutation.

Case Reports in Oncology

Singh Y[1], Bali C[2].

[1]Brampton, Ont., Canada.

[2]Ajax, Ont., Canada.

Abstract

Acute lymphoblastic leukemia (ALL) is a cancer of the white blood cells and is typically well treated with combination chemotherapy, with a remission state after 5 years of 94% in children and 30-40% in adults. To establish how aggressive the disease is, further chromosome testing is required to determine whether the cancer is myeloblastic and involves neutrophils, eosinophils or basophils, or lymphoblastic involving B or T lymphocytes. This case study is on a 14-year-old patient diagnosed with a very aggressive form of ALL (positive for the Philadelphia chromosome mutation). A standard bone marrow transplant, aggressive chemotherapy and radiation therapy were revoked, with treatment being deemed a failure after 34 months. Without any other solutions provided by conventional approaches aside from palliation, the family administered cannabinoid extracts orally to the patient. Cannabinoid resin extract is used as an effective treatment for ALL with a positive Philadelphia chromosome mutation and indications of dose-dependent disease control. The clinical observation in this study revealed a rapid dose-dependent correlation.

PubMed Link: https://www.ncbi.nlm.nih.gov/pubmed/24474921

"It is acknowledged that significant research needs to be conducted to reproduce these results and that in vitro studies cannot always be reproduced in clinical trials and the human physiological microenvironment. However, the numerous research studies and this particular clinical case are powerful enough to warrant implementing clinical trials to determine dose ranges, cannabinoid profiles and ratios, the methods of administration that produce the most efficacious therapeutic responses and the reproducibility of the results. It is tempting to speculate that, with integration of this care in a setting of full medical and laboratory support, a better outcome may indeed be achieved in the future."

Complete Study Link:

https://www.ncbi.nlm.nih.gov/pmc/articles/PMC3901602/

Inhibition of colon carcinogenesis by a standardized Cannabis sativa extract with high content of cannabidiol.

Phytomedicine.

Romano B[1], Borrelli F[2], Pagano E[2], Cascio MG[3], Pertwee RG[3], Izzo AA[4].

[1]Department of Pharmacy, University of Naples Federico II, Naples, Italy; Endocannabinoid Research Group, Italy; School of Medical Sciences, Institute of Medical Sciences, University of Aberdeen, Aberdeen AB25 2ZD, United Kingdom.

[2]Department of Pharmacy, University of Naples Federico II, Naples, Italy; Endocannabinoid Research Group, Italy.

[3]School of Medical Sciences, Institute of Medical Sciences, University of Aberdeen, Aberdeen AB25 2ZD, United Kingdom.

[4]Department of Pharmacy, University of Naples Federico II, Naples, Italy; Endocannabinoid Research Group, Italy.

Abstract:

PURPOSE:
Colon cancer is a major public health problem. Cannabis-based medicines are useful adjunctive treatments in cancer patients. Here, we have investigated the effect of a standardized Cannabis sativa extract with high content of cannabidiol (CBD), here named CBD BDS, i.e. CBD botanical drug substance, on colorectal cancer cell proliferation and in experimental models of colon cancer in vivo.
METHODS:
Proliferation was evaluated in colorectal carcinoma (DLD-1 and HCT116) as well as in healthy colonic cells using the MTT assay. CBD BDS binding was evaluated by its ability to displace [(3)H]CP55940 from human cannabinoid CB1 and CB2 receptors. In vivo, the effect of CBD BDS was examined on the preneoplastic lesions (aberrant crypt foci), polyps and tumours induced by the carcinogenic agent azoxymethane (AOM) as well as in a xenograft model of colon cancer in mice.
RESULTS:
CBD BDS and CBD reduced cell proliferation in tumoral, but not in healthy, cells. The effect of CBD BDS was counteracted by selective CB1 and CB2 receptor antagonists. Pure CBD reduced cell proliferation in a CB1-sensitive antagonist manner only. In binding assays, CBD BDS showed greater affinity than pure CBD for both CB1 and CB2 receptors, with pure CBD having very little affinity. In vivo, CBD BDS reduced AOM-induced preneoplastic lesions and polyps as well as tumour growth in the xenograft model of colon cancer.
CONCLUSIONS:
CBD BDS attenuates colon carcinogenesis and inhibits colorectal cancer cell proliferation via CB1 and CB2 receptor activation. The results may have some clinical relevance for the use of Cannabis-based medicines in cancer patients.

Cannabinoids as therapeutic agents in cancer: current status and future implications.
Oncotarget.

Chakravarti B[1], Ravi J[2], Ganju RK[3].

[1]Division of Endocrinology, Central Drug Research Institute, Lucknow, UP, India; These authors contributed equally to this work.

[2]Department of Pathology, The Ohio State University, Columbus, Ohio, USA; These authors contributed equally to this work.

[3]Department of Pathology, The Ohio State University, Columbus, Ohio, USA.

Abstract:

The pharmacological importance of cannabinoids has been in study for several years. Cannabinoids comprise of (a) the active compounds of the Cannabis sativa plant, (b) endogenous as well as (c) synthetic cannabinoids. Though cannabinoids are clinically used for anti-palliative effects, recent studies open a promising possibility as anti-cancer agents. They have been shown to possess anti-proliferative and anti-angiogenic effects in vitro as well as in vivo in different cancer models. Cannabinoids regulate key cell signaling pathways that are involved in cell survival, invasion, angiogenesis, metastasis, etc. There is more focus on CB1 and CB2, the two cannabinoid receptors which are activated by most of the cannabinoids. In this review article, we will focus on a broad range of cannabinoids, their receptor dependent and receptor independent functional roles against various cancer types with respect to growth, metastasis, energy metabolism, immune environment, stemness and future perspectives in exploring new possible therapeutic opportunities.

FROM FULL TEXT:

"One of the important aspects of an effective anti-tumor drug is its ability to inhibit proliferation of cancer cells. Cancer cells proliferate rapidly in uncontrolled manner. Also, these cells escape death mechanism which a normal cell undergoes like apoptosis. Apoptosis is a kind of programmed cell death (PCD) mechanism which involves activation of caspase dependent and independent pathways [39]. Cannabinoids have been proved to be anti-proliferative and apoptotic drugs. This section comprises of the detailed role of cannabinoids in modulation of tumor proliferation, cell cycle and apoptosis in various cancer types."

Complete Study Link:

Colon carcinogenesis is inhibited by the TRPM8 antagonist cannabigerol, a Cannabis-derived non-psychotropic cannabinoid.

Carcinogenesis.

Borrelli F[1], Pagano E[1], Romano B[1], Panzera S[1], Maiello F[2], Coppola D[2], De Petrocellis L[3], Buono L[3], Orlando P[4], Izzo AA[5].

[1]Department of Pharmacy, University of Naples Federico II, Via D. Montesano 49, 80131 Naples, Italy, Department of Diagnostic Services (Anatomy and Pathologic Histology Service), Ospedale dei Pellegrini, ASL 1, 80135 Naples, Italy, Institute of Biomolecular Chemistry, National Research Council, Via Campi Flegrei 34, 80078 Pozzuoli, Naples, Italy and Institute of Protein Biochemistry, National Research Council, Via P. Castellino 111, 80131 Naples, Italy.

[2]Department of Diagnostic Services (Anatomy and Pathologic Histology Service), Ospedale dei Pellegrini, ASL 1, 80135 Naples, Italy.

[3]Institute of Biomolecular Chemistry, National Research Council, Via Campi Flegrei 34, 80078 Pozzuoli, Naples, Italy and.

[4]Institute of Protein Biochemistry, National Research Council, Via P. Castellino 111, 80131 Naples, Italy.

[5]Department of Pharmacy, University of Naples Federico II, Via D. Montesano 49, 80131 Naples, Italy, Department of Diagnostic Services (Anatomy and Pathologic Histology Service), Ospedale dei Pellegrini, ASL 1, 80135 Naples, Italy, Institute of Biomolecular Chemistry, National Research Council, Via Campi Flegrei 34, 80078 Pozzuoli, Naples, Italy and Institute of Protein Biochemistry, National Research Council, Via P. Castellino 111, Naples, Italy

Abstract:
Cannabigerol (CBG) is a safe non-psychotropic Cannabis-derived cannabinoid (CB), which interacts with specific targets involved in carcinogenesis. Specifically, CBG potently blocks transient receptor potential (TRP) M8 (TRPM8), activates TRPA1, TRPV1 and TRPV2 channels, blocks 5-hydroxytryptamine receptor 1A (5-HT1A) receptors and inhibits the reuptake of endocannabinoids. Here, we investigated whether CBG protects against colon tumourigenesis. Cell growth was evaluated in colorectal cancer (CRC) cells using the 3-(4,5-dimethylthiazole-2-yl)-2,5-diphenyl tetrazolium bromide and 3-amino-7-dimethylamino-2-methylphenazine hydrochloride assays; apoptosis was examined by histology and by assessing caspase 3/7 activity; reactive oxygen species (ROS) production by a fluorescent probe; CB receptors, TRP and CCAAT/enhancer-binding protein homologous protein (CHOP) messenger RNA (mRNA) expression were quantified by reverse transcription-polymerase chain reaction; small hairpin RNA-vector silencing of TRPM8 was performed by electroporation. The in vivo antineoplastic effect of CBG was assessed using mouse models of colon cancer. CRC cells expressed TRPM8, CB1, CB2, 5-HT1A receptors, TRPA1, TRPV1 and TRPV2 mRNA. CBG promoted apoptosis, stimulated ROS production, upregulated CHOP mRNA and reduced cell growth in CRC cells. CBG effect on cell growth was independent from TRPA1, TRPV1 and TRPV2 channels activation, was further increased by a CB2 receptor

antagonist, and mimicked by other TRPM8 channel blockers but not by a 5-HT1A antagonist. Furthermore, the effect of CBG on cell growth and on CHOP mRNA expression was reduced in TRPM8 silenced cells. In vivo, CBG inhibited the growth of xenograft tumours as well as chemically induced colon carcinogenesis. CBG hampers colon cancer progression in vivo and selectively inhibits the growth of CRC cells, an effect shared by other TRPM8 antagonists. CBG should be considered translationally in CRC prevention and cure.

PubMed Link: https://www.ncbi.nlm.nih.gov/pubmed/25269802

FROM FULL TEXT:

"It is estimated that by 2030, the number of new cancer cases will increase by 70% worldwide mainly due to adoption of western lifestyle habits (1–3). Globally, colorectal cancer (CRC) is a major life-threatening disease representing the third most common cancer in men and the second most common cancer in women worldwide (1). The American cancer society in the USA estimates that the probability to develop CRC during the life is 5.17% for men and 4.78% for women and predicts that this type of cancer will cause ~50 830 deaths in 2013 (3,4). Although significant progress has been made in understanding CRC development through epidemiological, laboratory and clinical studies, this type of cancer continues to be a major public health problem in the USA and many other parts of the world. Accordingly, novel therapeutic approaches, including chemopreventive measures, are urgently needed (5).

The plant Cannabis sativa contains >100 phytocannabinoids that have been used for years for both recreational and medicinal purposes (6,7) and, at least some of them, are now candidates for new anticancer therapies (8). Beside a direct anticancer action, phytocannabinoids have demonstrated to attenuate several important side effects induced by chemotherapeutics (9–11). Phytocannabinoids include psychotropic compounds such as $\Delta 9$-tetrahydrocannabinol and many other non-psychotropic compounds of therapeutic interest, such as cannabigerol (CBG). CBG appears as a relatively low concentration intermediate in the plant, although recent breeding works have yielded Cannabis chemotypes expressing 100% of their phytocannabinoid content as CBG (12,13). Older and recent studies support analgesic, antierythemic, antibacterial, antidepressant and antihypertensive actions for CBG (8,14). Relevant to the present investigation, CBG has been proved to be cytotoxic in high dosage on human epithelioid carcinoma cells (15), to be effective against breast cancer (16) and to inhibit keratinocyte proliferation (17). Furthermore, CBG reduced experimental intestinal inflammation, which is relevant in view of the observation that the risk of developing neoplasia leading to CRC is significantly increased in ulcerative colitis patients (18,19). Pharmacodynamic studies have shown that CBG interacts with receptors/enzymes involved in carcinogenesis. Specifically, CBG is a weak partial agonist of cannabinoid (CB)1 and CB2 receptors (20), inhibits the reuptake of endocannabinoids (21), is a potent 5-HT1A antagonist (20) and may interact with transient receptor potential (TRP) channels. Among the TRP channels, CBG has been shown to be a TRPA1, TRPV1 and TRPV2 agonist and, importantly, a potent TRPM8 antagonist (21), a TRP channel known to be involved in the growth of tumoural cells (22–25). Here, we have (i) investigated the effect and the mode of action of CBG on colorectal carcinoma cells growth, (ii) evaluated its possible chemopreventive action in the azoxymethane (AOM) model of colon cancer and (iii) assessed its possible curative effect in the xenograft model of colon cancer."

Complete Study Link:
https://academic.oup.com/carcin/article-lookup/doi/10.1093/carcin/bgu205

2015

Phytocannabinoids for Cancer Therapeutics: Recent Updates and Future Prospects.
Current Medicinal Chemistry

Patil KR, Goyal SN, Sharma C, Patil CR, Ojha S[1].

[1]Department of Pharmacology and Therapeutics, College of Medicine and Health Sciences United Arab Emirates University, Al Ain, United Arab Emirates, UAE.

Abstract:
Phytocannabinoids (pCBs) are lipid-soluble phytochemicals present in the plant, Cannabis sativa L. and non-cannabis plants which have a long history in recreation and traditional medicine. The plant and the constituents isolated were central in the discovery of the endocannabinoid system (ECS), the most new target for drug discovery. The ECS includes two G-protein-coupled receptors; the cannabinoid receptors-1 and -2 (CB1 and CB2) for marijuana's psychoactive principle $\Delta(9)$-tetrahydrocannabinol ($\Delta(9)$-THC), their endogenous small lipid ligands; namely anandamide (AEA) and 2-arachidonoylglycerol (2-AG), also known as endocannabinoids and the enzymes for endocannabinoid biosynthesis and degradation such as fatty acid amide hydrolase (FAAH) and monoacylglycerol lipase (MAGL). The ECS has been suggested as a pro-homeostatic and pleiotropic signaling system activated in a time- and tissue-specific way during pathological conditions including cancer. Targeting the CB1 receptors becomes a concern because of adverse psychotropic reactions. Hence, targeting the CB2 receptors or the endocannabinoid metabolizing enzymes by pCBs obtained from plants lacking psychotropic adverse reactions has garnered interest in drug discovery. These pCBs derived from plants appear safe and effective with a wider access and availability. In the recent years, several pCBs derived other than non-cannabinoid plants have been reported to bind to and functionally interact with cannabinoid receptors and appear promising candidate for drug development including cancer therapeutics. Several of them also targets the endocannabinoid metabolizing enzymes that control endocannabinoid levels. In this article, we summarize and critically discuss the updates and future prospects of the pCBs as novel and promising candidates for cancer therapeutics.

PubMed Link: https://www.ncbi.nlm.nih.gov/pubmed/26179998

Proapoptotic effect of endocannabinoids in prostate cancer cells.

Oncology Reports

Orellana-Serradell O[1], Poblete CE[1], Sanchez C[1], Castellón EA[1], Gallegos I[2], Huidobro C[3], Llanos MN[4], Contreras HR[1].

[1]Physiology and Biophysics Program, Institute of Biomedical Sciences, Faculty of Medicine, University of Chile, Santiago, Chile.

[2]Pathological Anatomy Service, Clinic Hospital of the University of Chile, Santiago, Chile.

[3]Urology Service, Clinic Hospital of the University of Chile, Santiago, Chile.

[4]Laboratory of Nutrition and Metabolic Regulation, INTA, University of Chile, Santiago, Chile.

Abstract:

In the early stages, prostate cancer is androgen- dependent; therefore, medical castration has shown significant results during the initial stages of this pathology. Despite this early effect, advanced prostate cancer is resilient to such treatment. Recent evidence shows that derivatives of Cannabis sativa and its analogs may exert a protective effect against different types of oncologic pathologies. The purpose of the present study was to detect the presence of cannabinoid receptors (CB1 and CB2) on cancer cells with a prostatic origin and to evaluate the effect of the in vitro use of synthetic analogs. In order to do this, we used a commercial cell line and primary cultures derived from prostate cancer and benign prostatic hyperplasia. The presence of the CB1 and CB2 receptors was determined by immunohistochemistry where we showed a higher expression of these receptors in later stages of the disease (samples with a high Gleason score). Later, treatments were conducted using anandamide, 2-arachidonoyl glycerol and a synthetic analog of anandamide, methanandamide. Using the MTT assay, we proved that the treatments produced a cell growth inhibitory effect on all the different prostate cancer cultures. This effect was demonstrated to be dose-dependent. The use of a specific CB1 receptor blocker (SR141716) confirmed that this effect was produced primarily from the activation of the CB1 receptor. In order to understand the MTT assay results, we determined cell cycle distribution by flow cytometry, which showed no variation at the different cell cycle stages in all the cultures after treatment. Treatment with endocannabinoids resulted in an increase in the percentage of apoptotic cells as determined by Annexin V assays and caused an increase in the levels of activated caspase-3 and a reduction in the levels of Bcl-2 confirming that the reduction in cell viability noted in the MTT assay was caused by the activation of the apoptotic pathway. Finally, we observed that endocannabinoid treatment activated the Erk pathway and at the same time, produced a decrease in the activation levels of the Akt pathway. Based on these results, we suggest that endocannabinoids may be a beneficial option for the treatment of prostate cancer that has become nonresponsive to common therapies.

PubMed Link: https://www.ncbi.nlm.nih.gov/pubmed/25606819

Complete Study:
https://www.ncbi.nlm.nih.gov/pmc/articles/PMC4358087/

Cannabis and cancer: reality or pipe dream?
The Lancet.Oncology

Paul Cathcart, Alex de Giorgio, Justin Stebbing
Imperial College, London, UK.

Abstract:
Among alternative cancer treatments, cannabis inhabits a peculiarly politicised position, hailed as a suppressed panacea by some, denounced as a psychosis-inducing and illegal drug by others. In the middle ground, there is a growing acceptance of the plant's capacity for effective pain and nausea relief, and even tentative suggestions of potentiation of treatments such as chemotherapy and even direct action to restrain tumour cells by various routes. The doctor is immediately put in a compromising position: legally forbidden from advocating use, but professionally bound to ease suffering to the best of their abilities.

PubMed Link: https://www.ncbi.nlm.nih.gov/pubmed/26433817

Complete Study:
http://www.thelancet.com/journals/lanonc/article/PIIS1470-2045%2815%2900302-2/abstract

The Antitumor Activity of Plant-Derived Non-Psychoactive Cannabinoids.
Journal of Neuroimmune Pharmacology

McAllister SD[1], Soroceanu L, Desprez PY.

[1] California Pacific Medical Center Research Institute, 475 Brannan Street, San Francisco, CA, USA

Abstract:
As a therapeutic agent, most people are familiar with the palliative effects of the primary psychoactive constituent of Cannabis sativa (CS), $\Delta(9)$-tetrahydrocannabinol (THC), a molecule active at both the cannabinoid 1 (CB1) and cannabinoid 2 (CB2) receptor subtypes. Through the activation primarily of CB1 receptors in the central nervous system, THC can reduce nausea, emesis and pain in cancer patients undergoing chemotherapy. During the last decade, however, several studies have now shown that CB1 and CB2 receptor agonists can act as direct antitumor agents in a variety of aggressive cancers. In addition to THC, there are many other cannabinoids found in CS, and a majority produces little to no psychoactivity due to the inability to activate cannabinoid receptors. For example, the second most abundant cannabinoid in CS is the non-psychoactive cannabidiol (CBD). Using animal models, CBD has been shown to inhibit the progression of many types of cancer including glioblastoma (GBM), breast, lung, prostate and colon cancer. This review will center on mechanisms by which CBD, and other plant-derived cannabinoids inefficient at activating cannabinoid receptors, inhibit tumor cell viability, invasion, metastasis, angiogenesis, and the stem-like potential of cancer cells. We will also discuss the

181

ability of non-psychoactive cannabinoids to induce autophagy and apoptotic-mediated cancer cell death, and enhance the activity of first-line agents commonly used in cancer treatment.

PubMed Link: https://www.ncbi.nlm.nih.gov/pubmed/25916739

2016

Ligands for cannabinoid receptors, promising anticancer agents.
Life Sciences

Nikan M[1], Nabavi SM[2], Manayi A[3].

[1]Medicinal Plants Research Center, Faculty of Pharmacy, Tehran University of Medical Sciences, Tehran, Iran.

[2]Applied Biotechnology Research Center, Baqiyatallah University of Medical Sciences, Tehran, Iran.

[3]Medicinal Plants Research Center, Faculty of Pharmacy, Tehran University of Medical Sciences, Tehran, Iran.

Abstract:

Cannabinoid compounds are unique to cannabis and provide some interesting biological properties. These compounds along with endocannabinoids, a group of neuromodulator compounds in the body especially in brain, express their effects by activation of G-protein-coupled cannabinoid receptors, CB1 and CB2. There are several physiological properties attributed to the endocannabinoids including pain relief, enhancement of appetite, blood pressure lowering during shock, embryonic development, and blocking of working memory. On the other hand, activation of endocannabinoid system may be suppresses evolution and progression of several types of cancer. According to the results of recent studies, CB receptors are over-expressed in cancer cell lines and application of multiple cannabinoid or cannabis-derived compounds reduce tumor size through decrease of cell proliferation or induction of cell cycle arrest and apoptosis along with desirable effect on decrease of tumor-evoked pain. Therefore, modulation of endocannabinoid system by inhibition of fatty acid amide hydrolase (FAAH), the enzyme, which metabolized endocannabinoids, or application of multiple cannabinoid or cannabis-derived compounds, may be appropriate for the treatment of several cancer subtypes. This review focuses on how cannabinoid affect different types of cancers.

In vitro and in vivo efficacy of non-psychoactive cannabidiol in neuroblastoma.

Current Oncology (Toronto, Ontario)

Fisher T[1], Golan H[2], Schiby G[3], PriChen S[4], Smoum R[5], Moshe I[1], Peshes-Yaloz N[6], Castiel A[6], Waldman D[2], Gallily R[7], Mechoulam R[5], Toren A[8].

[1]Pediatric Hemato-Oncology Research Laboratory, Sheba Cancer Research Center.

[2]Pediatric Hemato-Oncology Research Laboratory, Sheba Cancer Research Center; Department of Pediatric Hemato-Oncology, The Edmond and Lily Safra Children's Hospital.

[3]Department of Pathology, The Chaim Sheba Medical Center, Tel-Hashomer, Israel;

[4]Pediatric Stem Cell Research Institute, The Chaim Sheba Medical Center, Tel-Hashomer, Israel;

[5]Institute for Drug Research, Hebrew University of Jerusalem, Jerusalem, Israel;

[6]Cancer Research Center, The Chaim Sheba Medical Center, Tel-Hashomer, Israel;

[7]The Lautenberg Center for General and Tumour Immunology, Hebrew University of Jerusalem, Jerusalem, Israel;

[8]Department of Pediatric Hemato-Oncology, The Edmond and Lily Safra Children's Hospital; Sackler School of Medicine, Tel-Aviv University, Tel-Aviv, Israel.

Abstract:
BACKGROUND:
Neuroblastoma (nbl) is one of the most common solid cancers in children. Prognosis in advanced nbl is still poor despite aggressive multimodality therapy. Furthermore, survivors experience severe long-term multi-organ sequelae. Hence, the identification of new therapeutic strategies is of utmost importance. Cannabinoids and their derivatives have been used for years in folk medicine and later in the field of palliative care. Recently, they were found to show pharmacologic activity in cancer, including cytostatic, apoptotic, and antiangiogenic effects.
METHODS:
We investigated, in vitro and in vivo, the anti-nbl effect of the most active compounds in Cannabis, $\Delta(9)$-tetrahydrocannabinol (thc) and cannabidiol (cbd). We set out to experimentally determine the effects of those compounds on

viability, invasiveness, cell cycle distribution, and programmed cell death in human nbl SK-N-SH cells.

RESULTS:

Both compounds have antitumourigenic activity in vitro and impeded the growth of tumour xenografts in vivo. Of the two cannabinoids tested, cbd was the more active. Treatment with cbd reduced the viability and invasiveness of treated tumour cells in vitro and induced apoptosis (as demonstrated by morphology changes, sub-G1 cell accumulation, and annexin V assay). Moreover, cbd elicited an increase in activated caspase 3 in treated cells and tumour xenografts.

CONCLUSIONS:

Our results demonstrate the antitumourigenic action of cbd on nbl cells. Because cbd is a nonpsychoactive cannabinoid that appears to be devoid of side effects, our results support its exploitation as an effective anticancer drug in the management of nbl.

PubMed Link: https://www.ncbi.nlm.nih.gov/pubmed/27022310

Cannabis and Cancer: Toward a New Understanding
Current Oncology
M.A. Ware, MBBS MSc
Anesthesia and Family Medicine, McGill University, and the Alan Edwards Pain Management Unit, McGill University Health Centre, Montreal, QC.

The treatment of cancer, including the disease itself and the symptoms associated with cancer and its therapy, is one of the most important emerging frontiers in cannabinoid therapeutics. With new regulatory environments opening up in Canada and around the world, access to a variety of quality-controlled cannabis-based products and administration techniques is becoming a reality for patients and their families desperate for new approaches to the devastating effects of cancer. The same is true for scientists and clinical researchers, who are starting to realize that, after years of deep freeze on cannabis-related research, funding, and materials, a thaw is starting. The promise, and even the hype, can reach hysterical proportions, with claims of cannabis cancer cures circulating in cyberspace at a furious pace. The challenge in the coming months and years will be to channel this interest into a productive clinical research program that informs and enlightens all those affected by cancer and its ravages.

Cannabinoids for Symptom Management and Cancer Therapy: The Evidence.

Journal of National Comprehensive Cancer Network
Davis MP.

From Cleveland Clinic Lerner School of Medicine, Case Western University, and Palliative Medicine and Supportive Oncology Services, Division of Solid Tumor, Taussig Cancer Institute, The Cleveland Clinic, Cleveland, Ohio.

Abstract (edited):
"Multiple cancers express cannabinoid receptors directly related to the degree of anaplasia and grade of tumor. Preclinical in vitro and in vivo studies suggest that cannabinoids may have anticancer activity. Paradoxically, cannabinoid receptor antagonists also have antitumor activity."

Cannabidiol rather than Cannabis sativa extracts inhibit cell growth and induce apoptosis in cervical cancer cells.

BMC Complementary and Alternative Medicine
Lukhele ST, Motadi LR.
Department of Biochemistry, North-west University (Mafikeng campus), Potchefstroom, South Africa.

Abstract:
BACKGROUND:
Cervical cancer remains a global health related issue among females of Sub-Saharan Africa, with over half a million new cases reported each year. Different therapeutic regimens have been suggested in various regions of Africa, however, over a quarter of a million women die of cervical cancer, annually. This makes it the most lethal cancer amongst black women and calls for urgent therapeutic strategies. In this study we compare the anti-proliferative effects of crude extract of Cannabis sativa and its main compound cannabidiol on different cervical cancer cell lines.
METHODS:
To achieve our aim, phytochemical screening, MTT assay, cell growth analysis, flow cytometry, morphology analysis, Western blot, caspase 3/7 assay, and ATP measurement assay were conducted.
RESULTS:

Results obtained indicate that both cannabidiol and Cannabis sativa extracts were able to halt cell proliferation in all cell lines at varying concentrations. They further revealed that apoptosis was induced by cannabidiol as shown by increased subG0/G1 and apoptosis through annexin V. Apoptosis was confirmed by overexpression of p53, caspase 3 and bax. Apoptosis induction was further confirmed by morphological changes, an increase in Caspase 3/7 and a decrease in the ATP levels.

CONCLUSIONS:

In conclusion, these data suggest that cannabidiol rather than Cannabis sativa crude extracts prevent cell growth and induce cell death in cervical cancer cell lines.

PubMed Link: https://www.ncbi.nlm.nih.gov/pubmed/27586579

Complete Study Links:
https://www.ncbi.nlm.nih.gov/pmc/articles/PMC5009497/
https://www.ncbi.nlm.nih.gov/pmc/articles/PMC5009497/pdf/12906_2016_Article_1280.pdf

2017

Cannabidiolic acid-mediated selective down-regulation of c-fos in highly aggressive breast cancer MDA-MB-231 cells: possible involvement of its down-regulation in the abrogation of aggressiveness.

Journal of Natural Medicines

Takeda S[1,2], Himeno T[2], Kakizoe K[2], Okazaki H[2], Okada T[3], Watanabe K[4], Aramaki H[5,6].

[1]Laboratory of Xenobiotic Metabolism and Environmental Toxicology, Faculty of Pharmaceutical Sciences, Hiroshima International University (HIU), 5-1-1 Hiro-koshingai, Kure, Hiroshima, Japan.

[2]Department of Molecular Biology, Daiichi University of Pharmacy, 22-1 Tamagawa-cho, Minami-ku, Fukuoka, Japan.

[3]Biomedical Research Institute, National Institute of Advanced Industrial Science and Technology (AIST), 1-1-1, Higashi, Tsukuba, Ibaraki, Japan.

[4]Pharmaceutical Education Center, Daiichi University of Pharmacy, 22-1 Tamagawa-cho, Minami-ku, Fukuoka, Japan.

[5]Department of Molecular Biology, Daiichi University of Pharmacy, 22-1 Tamagawa-cho, Minami-ku, Fukuoka, Japan.

[6]Drug Innovation Research Center, Daiichi University of Pharmacy, 22-1 Tamagawa-cho, Minami-ku, Fukuoka, Japan.

Abstract:

The physiological activities of cannabidiolic acid (CBDA), a component of fiber-type cannabis plants, have been demonstrated and include its function as a protector against external invasion by inducing cannabinoid-mediated necrosis (Shoyama et al., Plant Signal Behav 3:1111-1112, 2008). The biological activities of CBDA have been attracting increasing attention. We previously identified CBDA as an inhibitor of the migration of MDA-MB-231 cells, a widely used human breast cancer cell line in cancer biology, due to its highly aggressive nature. The chemical inhibition and down-regulation of cyclooxygenase-2 (COX-2), the expression of which has been detected in ~40 % of human invasive breast cancers, are suggested to be involved in the CBDA-mediated abrogation of cell migration. However, the molecular mechanism(s) responsible for the CBDA-induced down-regulation of COX-2 in MDA-MB-231 cells have not yet been elucidated. In the present study, we describe a possible mechanism by which CBDA abrogates the expression of COX-2 via the selective down-regulation of c-fos, one component of the activator protein-1 (AP-1) dimer complex, a transcription factor for the positive regulation of the COX-2 gene.

PubMed Link: https://www.ncbi.nlm.nih.gov/pubmed/27530354

Despite all of these studies, the United States government has yet to fund *one* human cannabis-cancer trial!
As of May, 2017

Many of your friends, and family will be touched by cancer at some point in their lives.

The majority of politicians, and physicians, are *unaware* of the preclinical evidence, and how human studies need to be performed.

This book attempts to bring this issue to the attention of everyone, to facilitate a change.

Consider sharing this book.

www.cureforcancerdelayed.com